CHAMPIONS FOR CHILDREN

The lives of modern child care pioneers

Revised edition

Bob Holman

This revised edition published in 2013

First edition published in Great Britain in 2001 by

The Policy Press
University of Bristol
Fourth Floor
Beacon House
Queen's Road
Bristol BS8 1QU
UK
Tel +44 (0)117 331 4054
Fax +44 (0)117 331 4093
e-mail tpp-info@bristol.ac.uk
www.policypress.co.uk

North American office:
The Policy Press
c/o The University of Chicago Press
1427 East 60th Street
Chicago, IL 60637, USA
t: +1 773 702 7700
f: +1 773-702-9756
e:sales@press.uchicago.edu
www.press.uchicago.edu

© Bob Holman 2013

British Library Cataloguing in Publication Data
A catalogue record for this book is available from the British Library.

Library of Congress Cataloging-in-Publication Data
A catalog record for this book has been requested.

ISBN 978 1 4473 0914 7 paperback
ISBN 978 1 86134 353 6 hardcover

Cover design by Robin Hawes
Front cover: image kindly supplied by www.alamy.com
Printed and bound in Great Britain by www.4edge.co.uk

Contents

Preface

The 1940s to 1960s could be called a golden age of child care: the 1940s witnessed public concern about children 'deprived of a normal home life', which led to the government establishing the first local authority service, the Children's Departments, to offer specialised help to such children. In the 1950s the employees of these departments struggled successfully to build up children's services. The 1960s were marked by a further expansion of the Children's Departments as their skilled staff were given even wider duties in regard to the children's own parents and to young offenders. The 1960s also witnessed studies which established the fact that family poverty had not been abolished by the welfare state.

The Children's Departments were founded and run by a remarkable set of people. Many of them outlasted the departments which were amalgamated into social services departments (social work departments in Scotland) by 1971. A few continue in active service until this very day. It appears to me that social work students now know very little about these champions for children. Some of these champions also backed social reformers who continued to highlight child poverty. The latter are also champions for children.

My intention in this book is to record and so preserve the characters and deeds of six of these champions. I could have chosen many more, had space allowed. The six selected represent politicians, campaigners, children's officers, writers and researchers. My choice is shaped by the fact that I have known or at least met these champions. The exception is Eleanor Rathbone, who died in 1946, but I consider her efforts to combat child poverty so important to the children of subsequent years that she had to have the initial chapter. Furthermore, I feel I almost knew Eleanor through our mutual friend, Margaret Simey.

At first glance, it might appear that the six champions divide into two groups: Eleanor Rathbone and Peter Townsend, who strove to abolish child poverty, and Marjory Allen, Barbara Kahan, John Stroud and Clare Winnicott, who developed services for children deprived of satisfactory lives with their own parents. In fact, there was always an overlap. Eleanor Rathbone witnessed abject poverty in Liverpool but later she became concerned about the quality of the home life of children whose fathers spent long periods away in the armed forces or the Merchant Navy. Marjory Allen was dismayed at the lack of personal care for children in children's homes, but she also noted that they suffered low material standards. Barbara

Kahan forged an effective Children's Department which improved the treatment of children in public care, but she also campaigned for a reduction in poverty which would allow more children to remain with their parents. John Stroud's career direction was shaped by the poverty he saw in India but it was expressed both in writing about and in serving children who were separated from their parents. Clare Winnicott was deeply stirred by the material suffering of children in the 1930s, yet her main contribution was to be in the training of child care officers. Peter Townsend is internationally recognised as a campaigner against child poverty but it is less well known that his own experiences as a child in a lone-parent family shaped his values. The six children's champions came from very different backgrounds and include a titled lady and wealthy politician plus the children of a railway worker, a Baptist minister, a local government official and an actress. Yet, from their varied lives, two themes appear in common. First, that central government had to accept responsibility for dealing with child poverty. It was not sufficient to leave it to employers, voluntary agencies or the charity of individuals. Second, that local government should be the provider of a high quality service for deprived children. This was not to dismiss the contribution of voluntary services, but was rather a recognition that only local authorities could ensure a coverage of such services throughout the country. These two themes will appear again and again throughout the book. They are not entirely separate, for the champions perceived that poverty was a major factor in undermining family life.

My original proposal for this book concerned just the notables in the first six chapters. However, I was persuaded to write something about my own lifetime in child care. I do so reluctantly, for I am a pygmy alongside these giants. However, I hope that my story will provide an overview of the developments in child care from the 1940s to the present, along with some suggestions as to where developments in child care might go in the future.

Acknowledgements

The manuscript of this book was completed on time and accepted by a publisher early in 2000. Then came the writer's nightmare. The publisher had cash flow problems and announced that publication was postponed indefinitely. Fortunately, The Policy Press came to the rescue and it has been a pleasure to work with its team, especially Dawn Louise Rushen.

I wish to thank a number of people – some of whom are also children's champions in their own right – who have allowed me to interview them about the subjects of the book. I thank Keith Bilton, David Donnison, Frank Field, Ruth Lister, Jean Packman, Roy Parker, Brian Roycroft, Margaret Simey, Daphne Statham, Nick Stroud, Daphne Stroud and Sylvia Watson. George and Janie Thomas and David Bull kindly wrote to me. I also thank Barbara Kahan and Peter Townsend for allowing me to interview them about themselves. Unfortunately, Barbara died in August 2000, but I am pleased that she saw and approved the chapter about herself, and Peter died in 2009. Joel Kanter kindly let me see some of his drafts about Clare and Donald Winnicott which he is preparing for publication. Gary Williams of the Qualitative Data Archival Resource Centre at Essex University was most helpful in making available to me material about Peter Townsend and, in particular, Paul Thompson's *Life Story Interview* with Peter. Terry Philpot the editor-in-chief of *Community Care*, Jane Tunstill of the University of London, Margaret Hogan of the National Institute for Social Work and Nicola Hilliard of the National Children's Bureau, were also a source of encouragement. Above all, I wish to thank Annette to whom I am glad to have been married for 49 years.

I can only hope that the 21st century will be graced with children's champions who possess the skills, compassion and commitment of the six described in these pages.

ONE

Eleanor Rathbone, 1872-1946

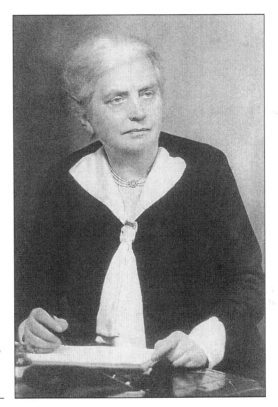

Photograph of Eleanor
Rathbone, kindly supplied by
University of Liverpool
Library, Special Collections
and Archives

She never had children, and never married. She came from a wealthy family and never lived alongside poor families. Yet she devoted much of her life to improving their material conditions by campaigning for children's allowances to be paid directly to mothers. The woman was Eleanor Rathbone and, just before she died, she contributed in the House of Commons to the enactment of the 1945 Family Allowances Act which, Hilary Land stated, "was probably the most notable personal triumph in legislation since the Act which celebrates the Plimsoll line" (Land, 1990, p

104). This chapter will attempt to trace how a privileged Victorian woman became a children's champion. Much of its content is drawn from an interview with Margaret Simey. Margaret was a friend of Eleanor Rathbone's and is now a distinguished elder stateswoman of social reform. In 1924, Margaret was one of the first degree students at Liverpool University in the School of Social Sciences, of which Eleanor was one of the founders. While there, Margaret went on placement to the Victoria Women's Settlement which was the base for much of Eleanor Rathbone's work. Thereafter, Margaret was associated with the same causes until Eleanor's death in 1946.

The Rathbone tradition

Eleanor Rathbone was born in 1872 to a family which was famous in Liverpool and beyond for its money and mercy. Her father, William Rathbone, multiplied the family fortunes in the China tea trade. A devoted Christian of the Unitarian church, he took seriously his duty to help others. Indeed, he regarded his money as something entrusted to him by God for the service of humankind. Later, when Eleanor wrote his biography, she called his life "a career of public usefulness" (Rathbone, 1905, p 493). It was a career helped by a tremendous drive, a kind of faith that almost anything could be achieved. He supported and founded charities in Liverpool, was a city councillor and then a Liberal MP. Married twice, William had eight sons and three daughters. The expectation was that his sons would take over their father's many roles. However, the sons never lived up to the standards he set in business and social life and, as Eleanor grew up, so her father increasingly prepared her to take on his charitable and political mantles.

They were mantles which Eleanor readily put on. Although she never identified with Christianity in the way that her father had, Eleanor believed that it was a heritage from him to use both her material and personal resources to benefit society. Margaret Simey wrote that her sense of social obligation was so sharp as "to be almost literally painful" (Simey, 1974, p 5). The direction she took led to some conflict with her mother, Emily. Emily Rathbone was no Victorian doormat and had encouraged Eleanor to develop wide interests as she was educated at home. Nonetheless, she expected Eleanor to marry and, as Susan Pedersen explains in an article which informs this and the following paragraph, insisted that, at the age of 18, she should enter "the marriage market of the London season" (Pedersen, 1996).

Despite her lack of formal education, Eleanor was clearly very intelligent and wanted to go to university. Her father was enthusiastic, her mother less so. She proceeded in 1893 to study philosophy at Somerville College, Oxford. Here she "found a group of liberal dons eager to win a new female audience for their philosophical creed of redemption through social service, and a community of single women able to offer the emotional sustenance she had been so long without" and she returned to the family home in 1896 "committed to the single life and able to cast her own quest for independence as part of a broader imperative towards selfless female action" (Pederson, 1996). Margaret Simey said, "Eleanor was not anti-men, just anti-marriage" and explained to me that Eleanor was not prepared to undergo the restrictions placed on women by Victorian marriage (Simey, 1999, interview with author). She also pointed out the influence on Eleanor, at this time, of Professor John MacCunn, a Scot who had come to Liverpool University as Professor of Moral Philosophy in 1881. MacCunn taught that for anyone to have to live a life of poverty and squalor was an offence against their dignity as citizens and a waste of their potential. It was the duty of other citizens to emancipate the poor, both for their own sake and for the good of society. He declared in a public lecture that "the purpose of social work is to emancipate the poor from oppression" (Simey, 1999, interview). MacCunn had faith in all people, in the potential of poor people and in the abilities of others to bring about change. His beliefs reinforced and enlarged the philosophy of Eleanor Rathbone.

Early activities

William persuaded his daughter both to volunteer as a friendly visitor for the Central Relief Society and also to undertake a study of one of his great concerns, the nature and effects of casual labour in the docks. By the time William died in 1902, Eleanor was establishing her own ideas. She was not impressed with the amateurish approach of some of the visitors at the Central Relief Society and gravitated to the Victoria Women's Settlement, founded in 1897 with, almost inevitably, two Rathbones on the committee. Here she met its young warden, Elizabeth Macadam. Mary Stocks, a close colleague of Eleanor and author of her biography, commented, "Elizabeth Macadam became in due course the friend and companion of Eleanor's existence until death did them part, and at no subsequent period was Eleanor lonely" (Stocks, 1949, p 58). Eleanor became the Settlement's honorary secretary and with Elizabeth they built it up as a centre for women's work, social activity and social work training.

Margaret Simey believes that the Settlement was crucial to Eleanor for, in a male-dominated city, it became a place where women could work together.

The study of dock labour was issued in 1903 as *Conditions of labour at the Liverpool Docks* (Rathbone, 1903). It was the first of Eleanor's many publications. It focused on the inefficiency of, and hardship involved in, a system whereby dockers had to assemble each week in the hope that employers would take them on. The study was also important to Eleanor for four other reasons. First, she established the method by which she painstakingly collected reliable data on which she based her conclusions and recommendations. Second, it brought her face-to-face with the unemployment, the overcrowding, the ill-health and the social deprivations of many citizens; henceforth, poverty was to be one of her central concerns. Third, it showed her that the effects of unemployment and irregular employment were felt most keenly by mothers and their children. Finally, it taught her that poverty was not due largely to individual defects, to an inability to be thrifty, but rather to wages that were too low and unemployment that was too frequent.

In 1909, Eleanor followed her father into politics and was elected as an Independent to Liverpool City Council. She was the first woman to be elected and was committed to social reform. The time was right for her. She had outstanding abilities and was dedicated to public service. Yet, if she had been born just a few years earlier she could not have attended Oxford University (which was closed to non-conformists until 1871), and could not have been an elected representative. The time was also ripe in that poverty, especially that of children, was widespread and required someone to establish that new methods were needed to counter it. When she was elected councillor, Eleanor was 37, with her best years yet to come.

Women and poverty

Eleanor Rathbone's focus on the nature and effects of poverty on women and children were highlighted by a series of further studies. The Victoria Women's Settlement, the Liverpool Women's Industrial Council and four other bodies combined to investigate the domestic conditions of dock labourers. Eleanor took a major part in a study which examined less the wages of the men and more the housekeeping money of their wives. Four hundred and twenty-nine women recorded their budgets for four weeks. Published in 1909 as *How the casual labourer lives* (Rathbone, 1909), it showed that two thirds of the families were living below the stringent poverty line which Seebohm Rowntree had used in his York research (Rowntree, 1901). They mostly lived in poor housing conditions, had inadequate diets, and were prone to ill-health. Eleanor also examined the incomes of women employed in cigar making and became convinced that women workers were so badly paid that wages alone would not take them out of poverty. From these and other investigations she came to some important conclusions.

In contrast to much contemporary opinion, Eleanor Rathbone was convinced that generally poverty was not due to personal inadequacy, ignorance or fecklessness. Indeed, she began to admire the economic capabilities of poor mothers and to resent the criticism made of them by the affluent. She declared:

> If the well-to-do people who enlarge on the incompetence of the English working woman and undertake to teach her 'Mothercraft' had to lead her life under her conditions, how many of them could stand the strain for a week? (cited in Alberti, 1996, p 35)

Further, Eleanor began to assert that the state would have to accept more responsibility for the relief of poverty and for deciding what was the minimum income below which no citizen's income should drop.

Given her doubts that increased women's wages were the answer – partly because most mothers could not work, partly because trades unions as well as political parties were opposed to the concept of equal pay for women, and partly because even most women seemed uninterested – she looked for alternatives. The idea of paying an endowment or allowance for children did not originate with Eleanor Rathbone – methodist ministers had received allowances for their children since the time of Wesley. But it was Eleanor Rathbone who was to spearhead the campaign for the state to pay an allowance. Before embarking on that campaign, however, she became involved in a direct and practical experiment.

The Liverpool Women's Industrial Council investigated the plight of the wives of seamen. As its members expected, it was revealed that many seamen did not make provision for their families before they left for sea with the consequence that wives were often driven into the grasp of ruthless moneylenders. The Industrial Council, with Eleanor prominent, won the support of the social scientist, Charles Booth, and the Liverpool MP, Richard Holt, both of whom had shipping interests. The outcome was legislation which allowed shipping firms to make 'allotments' of wages to the wives providing the husbands requested it. In Holt's own shipping company, 90% did so with the result that the sufferings of families were much reduced.

Eleanor's next battle proved much harder. Her growing reputation was such that in 1907 she had been invited to give evidence to the Royal Commission on the Poor Laws. She focused particularly on the low rates of Poor Law out-relief to widows and their children. She argued that it was not the mothers' fault that they had been widowed, that they were doing a valuable job in looking after their children, and that their income should be more in line with what they would have received from their husbands. Both the Majority and Minority Reports of the Commission were swayed by her arguments and in 1909 it was recommended that the rates for widows be raised. The Liverpool Board of Guardians, however, was not moved even when Eleanor and her colleagues produced case histories of the material plight of local widows. Clearly, if poverty was to be tackled it could not depend on the vagaries of local Poor Law boards. It took the First World War to give impetus to the case for more state intervention. It was the events of the war which also had positive implications for one of Eleanor's other great passions: women's suffrage.

Simultaneously with her social work and social reform activities, Eleanor sided with feminists in their struggle for the vote. She was of the non-militant variety and soon became secretary of the Liverpool Women's Suffrage Society and, from 1900, was on the executive of the National Union of Women's Suffrage Societies, which later became the National Union of Societies for Equal Citizenship. Given the focus of this book, however, little can be said in this chapter about her struggle to obtain equality for women. As Johanna Alberti shows (1996), it took up much of her time and emotions and involved her in a number of internal differences about methods and tactics. Eleanor Rathbone believed women should have the vote simply because they were as much a part of humanity as men. Margaret Simey said:

> Eleanor was not motivated by feminism. Feminism was the outcome. It affected her dreadfully that people down in the docks and others were not able to play their part in society, to fulfil their social obligations even though they wanted to be good citizens. This pushed her into child allowances, into politics and into the women's movement. The women's movement was the end product, she did not start with it. (Simey, 1999, interview with author)

Eleanor argued that women could only influence national decisions, especially those which determined whether or not poverty was tackled, if they had the vote and if they were represented in parliament. She added that most women would only be free to participate in political and social activities when they had incomes independent of their husbands' wages.

Whatever the precise reasons for her involvement, Eleanor also gained emotionally from the women's movement. As Alberti put it, "The suffrage movement brought together her sense of solidarity among women and the exhilaration she experienced in exercising the power of persuasion" (Alberti, 1996, p 30). She found friendships and fellowship with other women of like purpose which both met her emotional needs and also re-charged her batteries for her enormous workload.

The First World War (1914-18)

Eleanor Rathbone was not a pacifist. She was a patriot who, in both world wars, considered her country had to fight. By this period she was also a well-known public figure. She had a striking appearance and Mary Stocks wrote of her "remarkably fine eyes and that suggestion of eighteenth century dignity which prematurely white hair gives to unlined faces" (Stocks, 1949, p 59). She was poised to use the events of the war to strengthen the social causes in which she believed.

At the start of the war, the government announced that separation allowances would be paid to the wives and dependants of soldiers and sailors. Eleanor was pleased that the state recognised that it had an obligation to ensure that wives had money in their purses. Unfortunately, the state had no administrative machinery to pay the allowances. Voluntary bodies had to step into the breach. In Liverpool, where at least 35,000 men were in the armed forces, it was none other than Eleanor Rathbone who took over the Liverpool branch of the Soldiers' and Sailors' Family Association, recruited around a thousand voluntary workers, and set up dozens of district offices. Eleanor was soon criticising the level of allowances and the way in which assessments were calculated. Nonetheless, she regarded the innovation of allowances as a turning point. It recognised the importance of women in their role as mothers, and conceded that they should have payments made straight to them, not via their husbands. It was successful in that working wives and children were healthier in war time because they were getting a fair share of family income. Moreover, she argued that the allowances were of psychological benefit to women as they felt a greater sense of being valued by the state and had greater control over their circumstances. Indeed, she described it as "the greatest experiment that the world has ever seen in the State endowment of poverty" (cited in Alberti, 1996, p 40). Allowances were just one example of the extension of state action during these years. Whole industries became subject to state control. Again, Eleanor, although never a member of a socialist party, was quick to take up the argument that, if state intervention was justified to preserve the well-being of the nation in war time, so it would be justified to overcome poverty in peace time.

As the war proceeded, the army authorities expressed anxieties about the poor physical shape of many potential recruits. Eleanor was quick to point out that their ill-health derived from being brought up in poverty. She declared that by "doing just enough to keep slum babies alive but not enough to keep them healthy ... we are as a nation recruiting the national stock in increasing proportion from those who have sunk into the lowest strata because they are physically, mentally and morally degenerate" (cited in Alberti, 1996, p 38). These class-ridden words ring almost offensively today. But they were attuned to a nation at war and Eleanor had perceived a new and more powerful argument against poverty: the country needed healthy children at all times. Henceforth she campaigned for children as much as for mothers.

With her arguments and experience strengthened, in 1917 Eleanor founded the Family Endowment Committee (later the Family Endowment Society). A year later, the Committee, including Mary Stocks, was demanding that a weekly allowance be paid direct to all mothers for themselves and their children.

At the close of the war, the government conceded votes to women aged over 30. In 1918, Eleanor moved to London, partly to be with Elizabeth Macadam who had moved there, partly to be near the heart of government in order to campaign more effectively for social reform. Soon after, she was offered an OBE on the grounds of her services during the war. Unlike those who accept such honours by protesting that they do it on behalf of all their colleagues, Eleanor simply refused it. Later, it is believed she turned down a seat in the House of Lords. She never sought personal status.

The disinherited family

The elation at the end of the war was followed by years of anti-climax. In the 1918 General Election, all the women candidates were defeated (except for one Sinn Féin member who refused to take her seat). The National Union of Societies for Equal Citizenship, of which she was to become president, had severe divisions, particularly between those who wanted to concentrate on achieving equal pay for women and those who wanted priority for family endowments. But setbacks and disappointments never stopped Eleanor Rathbone. She had an inner conviction that what she was doing was ethically correct and she persisted. It was during these years that she wrote the clearest and most powerful case for family endowments (or family allowances, as they became known).

The disinherited family was published in 1924 (Rathbone, 1924). Eleanor argued that the family was an economic as well as a social institution. Families were consumers whose expenditure fuelled much economic activity. But, further, wives, in looking after male workers, and mothers, in raising future workers, were vital to the economic health of a nation. However, she continued, wives and mothers received no set income for these roles. Instead, they were entirely dependent on what their husbands gave them and, as this was often insufficient, the system weakened the institution of the family. In addition, she pointed out that the wages paid to men did not take into account the needs of their wives and children. Consequently, those with the smallest families could afford the best houses while those with the largest families were often found with inadequate diets in overcrowded homes. The solution put forward by Eleanor was that women required some form of income for themselves and their children which was both independent of the economic market and also independent of their husbands: family allowances.

In proposing a direct payment to women, Eleanor pointed out that she was not making a wild new suggestion as such schemes already existed in some other countries. She dryly commented that abroad the scheme had not destroyed family life, nor had it led to vast over-population as women bore babies just to get an allowance. She then proceeded to undermine the argument of her opponents that an allowance would harm the family by reducing its sense of responsibility, in that the family would become too dependent on state handouts. Poverty, she wrote, often led to evictions and people turning to the Poor Law which imposed on families such stringent conditions – often separating parents and children – that families were completely destroyed. This was state irresponsibility.

Eleanor did not want to keep women tied to the home. Nonetheless, she asserted that motherhood was one of society's most valuable tasks. She did not glamorise housework and baby care. Indeed, as she liked to point out, childbirth was four times as dangerous as working in a coal mine. She claimed that creating loving homes and raising healthy children were essential to the nation and therefore worthy of financial support.

She acknowledged that her scheme would cost up to £243 million a year but added that this had to be compared with over £260 million spent every year on tobacco, drink and amusements.

The disinherited family was the fullest and best plea for family endowments or allowances that had been published in Britain. Mary Stocks wrote about it in glowing terms, saying that it:

> ... is, in fact, one of the finest examples of polemical economic literature ever written. It has that rare combination of passionate conviction, intellectual grasp and terse literary exposition which one meets, for example, in Adam Smith's *Wealth of Nations*, in Tawney's *Acquisitive Society*, or in J. M. Keynes's *Economic Consequences of the Peace....* She conferred upon the family, as the most ancient institution known to human society and one of peculiar significance to women, a new status in the realm of economics. She brought to bear upon its problems a quality of analytical and constructive thought comparable to that which generations of penetrating male scholars had focused upon the problems of production, distribution and exchange. (Stocks, 1949, pp 96-7)

Nearly 50 years after Stocks, Frank Field MP stated that, with the book:

> She changed the debate about the distribution of income away from what she saw as an obsession with the distribution between classes, to one centring on differences between those households with and without children. And equally important, Eleanor was concerned about who got what within the family.... *The Disinherited Family* wins for her a place in 20th century economic classics, equal, I believe, to Keynes' *Employment, Income and Money*. In many passages her prose manages that of Keynes' scintillating style and she manages to express herself in a way that made algebraic equations redundant. (Field, 1996a)

The book provoked much opposition but was also widely praised as one of economic and social merit. In 1925, the National Union of Societies for Equal Citizenship passed a resolution in favour of a state scheme of family allowances. The book also succeeded in putting its subject on the public agenda, since it was widely discussed in the press. The next step was for Eleanor Rathbone to enter the public domain as a Member of Parliament.

Into parliament

In 1928, women won the vote on the same terms as men. A year later, Eleanor, age 57, was elected to parliament as the member for the Combined English Universities (a constituency which no longer exists) and remained an MP until her death. Despite her age she possessed the energy and drive of a much younger person. She did not have the wide-ranging constituency duties of most MPs and her private income enabled her to hire the kind of secretarial help then not available to many of her colleagues. She was therefore free to devote her time to the causes in which she believed. Frank Field, himself an MP, has written:

> Eleanor was one of the truly impressive parliamentarians of this century
> ... it is partly revealed by the examination of the entries under her name
> in Hansard's Index. Both the length of entries and the range of subject
> matters are truly staggering. (Field, 1996b)

It is worth adding that, until 1935, Eleanor also remained a local councillor in Liverpool, where she maintained her strong interest in housing conditions.

Eleanor was close to the Labour Party on most matters and frequently called for a redistribution of wealth and income from the rich to the poor. She was a reformist in the Fabian tradition and today might well have called herself an ethical socialist. But she did not join any political party and was glad to be called an Independent. In many ways her prime loyalties were to women rather than to party politics and she was always ready to speak on any issue which touched women. As Johanna Alberti has summed up:

> She was determined that women's presence in parliament should make
> a difference, and one way to do this was to call attention to such
> inequalities as the lack of provision for postgraduate women medical
> students; the lack of remunerative posts for women in post offices, and
> the treatment of women civil servants who did not get the same
> privileges as men. (Alberti, 1996, p 86)

She also pressed for more women to be placed on and to chair government bodies. In particular, she was concerned about the condition of women and their children. For instance, in 1932, legislation was introduced to cut back the health insurance benefits paid to married women to a lower rate than those of single women, which were already at a lower rate than those for men. In the House of Commons, she launched a sustained attack on the proposal. She saw the legislation as sexist, in that it discriminated unfairly between men and women, despite both being subject to sickness. Indeed, she argued that married women, by virtue of devoting themselves to families as well as work, were more likely to suffer ill-health than others.

Of all the vast range of subjects which she addressed, however, none received more of her attention than the poverty of millions of British families. Studies revealed continuing child poverty confirmed by another study in York by Seebohm Rowntree, where half the children suffered from nutritional deficiencies (Rowntree, 1941). She made the point that benefits in kind, such as school meals and milk, were not sufficient if parents lacked the money to feed families properly. Indeed, it was now the needs of poverty-stricken children that fuelled her campaign as much as the need to provide women with an independent income. She constantly pointed out that the levels of benefits awarded to unemployed and destitute people were not fixed according to their needs. Outside of parliament, she founded the Children's Minimum Council in 1934 to work for scales of unemployment benefit and assistance which were sufficient to allow families to purchase the diets recommended by the British Medical Association. Inside parliament, she called for government to establish what were minimum needs and then to set benefits so that no one would fall below them. Speaking in the Commons in 1934, she asked for benefits which "shall include a reasonable amount for rent and shall also include the minimum requirements of healthy physical subsistence" (cited in Alberti, 1996, p 172). Her pleas fell on deaf ears, for Britain was still in the throes of economic depression and politicians were more likely to cut benefits than to raise them.

It was now crystal clear to Eleanor that family allowances were the major means of relieving poverty. She had much persuasion to do. A number of Labour MPs were opposed, and in 1929 the General Council of the Trades Union Congress (TUC) came out against the allowances on the grounds that they would divide the interests of single and married men in wage negotiations, as well as providing employers with an excuse not to raise wages. Nonetheless, progress was made. She formed an all-party group of MPs who favoured family allowances. One member was James Griffiths who, as a Labour minister in post-war Britain, later oversaw the implementation of family allowances. Another was the Conservative, Leo Amery, who persuaded some private industrialists to include an allowance for children in their wage structures.

Eleanor did not restrict herself to Britain. One of the main forces driving her to stand for parliament was her passionate concern about the plight of women and children in India. Some Indian people, including Jawaharlal Nehru with whom she had a long correspondence when he was in prison, considered that she did not listen sufficiently to what Indians were saying, but there was no doubting her desire to help. She visited India, supported its movement for independence and campaigned for the rights of Indian women to be included in elected and appointed bodies.

She was also alert to the worsening diplomatic situation in Europe. Eleanor encouraged the government in its efforts to negotiate peace. At the same time, she considered that the country had a right to combat fascism and to defend democracy. As early as 1934, Eleanor was warning about Hitler and she was soon in the thick of trying to persuade the British authorities to accept refugees, especially Jewish refugees, from fascist regimes. Britain declared war against Germany in September 1939. Many citizens left London for safer places. Eleanor Rathbone refused to move even when the blitz was at its height. She continued her involvement with refugees and extended her concern to German and Italian nationals, many of them also refugees, who had been interned as 'aliens'. As honorary secretary of the Parliamentary Group on Refugees, she visited a camp at Huyton where thousands of internees were being detained in dreadful conditions. After the war, one of those internees recalled how they waited for her in the pouring rain:

> At last the door opens. A woman appears, behind her a man's face, both flanked by soldiers with fixed bayonets. The woman begins to address the men: 'You are not forgotten'.... They feel the warmth of her motherly face. The woman's face in the open door is beaten by the pouring rain. Her face, her voice are nursing the gleam of hope left in their hearts. (cited in Stocks, 1949, p 286)

And, true to her word, Eleanor Rathbone did get conditions improved and was able to get numbers released.

The 1945 Family Allowances Act

From 1939, vast numbers of children and young mothers were evacuated from the cities, which were expected to be bombed, to the countryside. These evacuations were to have a profound effect on services for deprived children (as will be explained in the next chapter) and on welfare services for all citizens, including the provision of state family allowances.

One immediate result of evacuation was to reveal the deficiencies of local authority welfare and health services in the areas to which the children and mothers were sent. Schools, day care facilities, welfare clinics, maternity services and hospitals were often unable to cope. As detailed elsewhere, central government had to intervene to ensure that local authorities had the resources to maintain services (Holman, 1995, ch 5). In short, the state acted to ensure that services were fairly distributed.

Most evacuated children were from working-class, often poor homes, from the huge urban inner cities. Many of the families who accepted them were prosperous and, if not, were certainly more used to healthy and stable environments. The reaction of the latter was initially one of disgust at the dirtiness, the manners and the habits of the children. Slowly the truth dawned that there was another Britain, a very deprived and neglected Britain. The social historian, Arthur Marwick, graphically put it:

> Ultimately, the significance of the evacuation experience was that it brought to middle- and upper-class households a consciousness for the first time of the deplorable conditions endemic in the rookeries and warrens which still existed in Britain's great industrial cities, and so, among the articulate few, aroused a new sense of social concern. In this sense evacuation was a unique experience and one of the most significant phenomena of the war. (Marwick, 1976, p 75)

Among the articulate few were several women's organisations of the kind Eleanor had supported. A number combined to form the Women's Group on Public Welfare which proceeded to study the conditions from which the evacuees had come. Its members were shocked by the 70,000 overcrowded houses in London, the high child mortality rates and the appalling poverty. They blamed not the individuals but the nation for these vast deprivations, and then listed urgent recommendations which included nursery education for all children, a national medical service, and children's allowances as the only way to tackle poverty. The findings were published in 1943 as *Our towns: A close-up* (Women's Group on Public Welfare, 1943). It soon sold out and was reprinted twice. Its significance was that state welfare was being advocated by middle-class women from the more conservative parts of Britain.

The evacuation was not the only factor which fuelled the demand for social reform. The war was as much a civilian war as an armed forces one. All kinds of people were being bombed, were suffering from shortages, were involved as fire fighters and air raid wardens. Not least, vast numbers of women were called on to take over men's jobs in their absence. As women began to see themselves as essential to the state, so they began to demand that the state treat them in a better fashion. Simultaneously, men in the armed forces abroad agitated to ensure that their families at home were not wanting for anything.

Eleanor Rathbone was not a woman to miss an opportunity. Soon after the war started, she was one of a group of MPs who sent a memorandum urging the government to introduce family allowances. She rapidly revised *The disinherited family* (1924) and published *The case for family allowances* (1940). She wrote that the war conditions heightened but did not create the case for family allowances. She pointed out that malnutrition, ill-health, bad housing and poverty existed in peace time as well as during war. She added, "The only thing that is new is the awakening sense of what these evils mean to the whole community" (Rathbone, 1940, p 106). In 1942 the TUC officially changed its stance and recommended that children's allowances be paid by the state on a non-contributory basis and unaccompanied by any means test. In the same year, William Temple, who was shortly to be Archbishop of Canterbury, was throwing his considerable influence behind increased state welfare. He declared that "family allowances perhaps in the form of food and clothes coupons having the value of money should be paid by the State to the mother for every child after the first two" (Temple, 1942, p 77).

Within the Commons, Eleanor also found that a number of trade unionist MPs were pressurising the government about the inadequacies of National Insurance payments for unemployed and sick workers. And now they were dealing not with a Conservative administration, but a coalition which included a number of ministers drawn from the Labour Party. One of them, Ernie Bevin, the Minister of Labour, appointed William Beveridge to undertake a far-ranging review. Eleanor was delighted because Beveridge had been converted to the concept of family allowances by her writings and, in 1924, when director of the London School of Economics, he had introduced a scheme of child allowances for staff. When the report appeared in 1942 as *The report on social insurance and allied services* (Beveridge, 1942), it proposed a comprehensive state insurance scheme, to which employers and employees would have to make contributions, and which would pay out benefits to meet needs associated with unemployment, disability, illness, retirement and widowhood. Crucially, the benefits would be given as a right and were not subject to a means test. Beveridge added that his scheme was based on the assumption that the government would also be introducing a national health service and family allowances. The report was a sell-out, with public reaction overwhelmingly in its favour (Beveridge, 1942).

Eleanor, of course, seized on the references to family allowances. Early in 1943, she headed a deputation to ask the Chancellor of the Exchequer for action. Within a few weeks, the government announced that it had accepted the principle of family allowances. Eleanor, within and without the Commons, then argued that they must be set at a level which would give women some financial independence, rather than at a low level which would just soothe a few consciences. When the Family Allowances Bill was introduced to the Commons in March 1945, she was disappointed that allowances were to start with the second child and that the amount per child was a mere five shillings, rather than the eight shillings mooted by Beveridge. But her anger was more aroused against the proposal that the money should be paid to the men. She threatened to vote against the Bill but did not have to do so in the end as it was amended in favour of women. John Macnicol asserts that family allowances became acceptable to policy makers less because of the arguments of Eleanor and her supporters and more because "they were seen as a means of enforcing work incentives, assisting labour mobility and concealing the problem of low pay" (Macnicol, 1980, p 217). Whether this was so or not, MPs gave the credit to Eleanor. When the Bill made its final passage through the Commons on 11 June 1945, speaker after speaker rose to acclaim it as her victory. She rejoiced in a victory that had established the principle and practice of family allowances. But she added that this was just the beginning of the fight and that the next round would be to raise the levels. Unfortunately, she was not to participate in the next round. She died suddenly on 2 January 1946, aged 73.

A complex character

This chapter is appreciative of Eleanor Rathbone's efforts on behalf of children and mothers. But she was not always applauded and not always liked, for she was a complex character. Politically, the very concept of family allowances drew fire from those who said it would undermine the unity and responsibility of families. Economically, it enraged some economists who claimed that the country could not afford to finance such allowances. She calmly responded to these arguments. Less easy to take were personal attacks such as the innuendoes about why she never married. In 1942, an MP declared in the Commons, "For years she has wasted her life advocating family allowances. I suppose that is a good enough substitute for the absence of a family" (cited in Alberti, 1996, p 142).

These attacks came from her political enemies. Other criticisms were voiced by those with whom she associated closely. There were feminists who considered she did not draw attention to women's unequal power position within the institution of marriage. As mentioned, some – her biographer and admirer Mary Stocks was one – thought that she failed to throw her weight behind the case for equal pay for women. Later feminists criticised her acceptance of the traditional family structure with its married couple: working husband with a wife who stayed at home to look after the children. Jane Lewis, in writing about Eleanor's "underlying conservatism", pointed out that she did not "wish allowances to go to unmarried mothers. Like many present day advocates of policies to support the family she had a clear idea of the kind of family she wished to be supported" (Lewis, 1983). There were socialists who felt that Eleanor, in concentrating on the women's movement, failed to understand the importance of class differences between women and that she accepted too easily the existing power of capitalism. There were some working-class activists who thought her approach somewhat patronising, in that she saw herself as doing good on behalf of the poor rather than with them. Eleanor's response to these criticisms was that of pragmatism. She considered that family allowances but not equal pay could be won in her lifetime. She recognised that capitalism was the cause of vast inequalities but, while others were waiting for the revolution, she would chip away for social reform. She accepted that she was a privileged, middle-class woman who spoke for others. Her justification was that the reforms she advocated would emancipate poor women so that they could control their own circumstances. Indeed, her anger was directed at so many middle-class women who, having won the vote, dropped out of political action.

Johanna Alberti points out that sometimes Eleanor's words contained a racist edge. She quotes from a speech, made by Eleanor in the Commons in 1935, in which she expresses British alarm about "the steady shrinkage of the white population compared with the yellow, the brown and the black" (cited in Alberti, 1996, p 139). This is not the only example of such sentiments and it cannot be denied that it implies a sense of white superiority. Yet the same Eleanor also acknowledged the great abilities of Asian women and passionately advocated that they be developed. She also supported moves towards self-government in British colonies by arguing that the "franchise and legal rights should be based upon the principle of equality for all without regard to race, colour, or sex" (cited in Alberti, 1996, p 171). Within Eleanor Rathbone there was a tension between a strong patriotism and a strong sense of equality. The former pushed her into statements which magnified the role of British people while the latter pulled her into the contradictory position in which she defended the value of all peoples.

At times, Eleanor came across as a very dominating person. Margaret Simey demurs at the word 'dominating'. Speaking about the Victoria Women's Settlement she said, "The place was dominated by Eleanor yet she was not a dominating person, although she was much larger than life. She was a Rathbone, rich, independent. She was unostentatious in the way that aristocrats are, they assume their superiority, they are accustomed to it" (Simey, 1999, interview with author). Certainly, she expected others to work as hard as she did and Mary Stocks wrote about one woman who kept ready a list of the meetings she had addressed for when Eleanor questioned her (Simey, 1999, interview). Certainly, people found it difficult to avoid the demands she made on them. Margaret Simey recalled that, when Eleanor wanted someone to chair the refugee work in Liverpool, "she fastened upon Tom [Margaret's husband] and once she fastened on you that was it. Our house became a centre for refugees" (Simey, 1999, interview).

Within parliament, her confidence in her own opinions and her readiness to interrupt those with whom she disagreed annoyed some members. Harold Nicolson wrote, after her death:

> Again and again I have observed Ministers or Under-Secretaries wince in terror when they observed that familiar figure advancing towards them along the corridors; they would make sudden gestures indicating that they had left some vital document behind them, swing round on their feet, and scurry back to their rooms. (cited in Stocks, 1949, p 142)

But, in the same passage, he also affectionately summed her up as a "fusion of ardour and selflessness" (cited in Stocks, 1949, p 142). At the same time, she possessed a tolerance which, for instance, insisted that the women's movement should unite varying strategies, militant and non-militant, and varying priorities. In short, she was very convinced of the correctness of her own views, very forceful in expressing them, very ready to argue them, and yet also very happy for others to put their case.

A forgotten champion

Within a few years of her death, Eleanor Rathbone's achievements had been largely forgotten, but not by everybody. Her surviving colleagues still remembered her. Margaret Simey said that, to the women who had gathered around her, she was "the example of what women could do. That put me into politics. In that group we had the first woman barrister in Liverpool, the first housing manager, a brilliant collection of women" (Simey, 1999, interview with author). Mary Stocks, a leading public figure for half a century, wrote that Eleanor was one of the three people who "were the principal influences in my life" (Stocks, 1970, p 47). Nonetheless, Eleanor Rathbone was not a name that came easily to the lips of later politicians, social workers and social reformers. Perhaps it was because she had no children to continue to uphold the Rathbone name. Perhaps because she never identified with any political party which could have placed her in its hall of heroes and heroines. Further, it must be said, Eleanor never sought fame or recognition. She lived modestly and never tried to impress others with her clothes or possessions. Mary Stocks points out that Eleanor never liked talking about herself and quotes from a letter which she wrote to Elizabeth Macadam in which she said, "I am not really any good at any form of social intercourse and nothing can cure that. And except when I am with you I am always alone to all intents and purposes" (cited in Stocks, 1949, p 181). Again, Margaret Simey explained that even though she was often with Eleanor, went to her home, campaigned for her, sat at her feet to learn, the relationship could never be described as a close friendship. She explained, "The relationship with Eleanor was always a working, purposeful one. We met for committees, for meetings, for campaigns" (Simey, 1999, interview). Further, Eleanor did not seek to be numbered with the mighty, did not want to be present at glittering occasions, did not attempt to secure social advancement by crawling after the establishment, and she wanted no honours. Yet one MP, Frank Field, has long regarded her as a great social reformer and, at last, in 1999, he succeeded in having her portrait unveiled in the House of Commons. Former colleagues like Margaret Simey, like-minded politicians such as Frank Field, and admiring feminists such as Johanna Alberti, are now managing to bring Eleanor back to public notice.

Oddly enough, although Eleanor did not seem to care what people thought about herself as an individual, and although she said she was not good at making social relationships, she cared passionately about individuals. Mary Stocks observed, "... the starting point of all her tireless activity was immediate compassion seen in terms of individual distress of body or mind.... But though her starting point was, I suppose, emotional, the action stimulated by emotion demanded hard thought and a meticulous marshalling and sifting of facts" (Stocks, 1970, pp 122-3). Margaret Simey recalled that, after Eleanor advertised for a shorthand typist, a black refugee turned up at her door. She could not type and her English was not very good but Eleanor immediately took her in and subsequently paid her fees to attend college, from which she obtained a job (Simey, 1999, interview with author). She was profoundly moved by individuals in poverty and she took up many individual cases. As Frank Field has put it, "She regarded each individual – at least if they were women and children – as sacred" (Field, 1996a). She was an individualist who did not fit into any political party, an individualist who could toe no party line because she wanted to select the causes for which she would campaign.

Once Eleanor started a campaign, she persisted until the end. She stayed with the women's movement through thick and thin. She helped refugees in the 1930s when the government was unsympathetic and right-wing groups were hostile. Her campaigning for family allowances extended over her lifetime. Her dogged endurance and refusal to accept defeat then served as an inspiration to others. Margaret Simey, speaking about both Eleanor Rathbone and Elizabeth Macadam, said, "The secret is that they were so consistent. They had a steady line, which at one time might emphasise education or housing, but which was always going straight ahead to emancipate the poor, black people, women, the Jews" (Simey, 1999, interview). She added, in writing, "To those who encountered her, it was as if she held the secret of perpetual inspiration" (Simey, 1974, p 15). Moreover, those who read about her are still inspired. Johanna Alberti wrote about her own experience of enduring years of reactionary government in Britain during the 1980s and early 1990s and continued, "This is very similar to the context in which Eleanor Rathbone lived and her energy has been a goad, her refusal to abandon hope an inspiration" (Alberti, 1996, p 5). Paradoxically, this insular, almost secretive, woman had the ability to strengthen those around her. This woman who wrote very little about herself still encourages others not to abandon their principles and objectives.

Above all, Eleanor Rathbone must retain a place in British social history as the author of family allowances. Of course, no person alone is ever responsible for a major piece of legislation, but it was Eleanor who kept the matter in the public eye for over 20 years. Her success, as Margaret Simey so well puts it, was "an astonishing achievement in face of the double handicap for a Member of Parliament of being a woman and belonging to no political party" (Simey, 1974, p 10). As Mary Stocks concluded, "If there had been no Eleanor ... there would have been no Family Allowances Act in 1945. It was *her* victory, conceived in her brain, brought to birth by her persistence, shaped by her vehemence" (Stocks, 1949, p 317). There can be little doubt that family allowances would have eventually become a part of Britain's welfare state. Eleanor Rathbone's contribution was to put them on the statute book earlier than would have been the case.

It is difficult to overestimate the importance of family allowances. Hilary Land writes, "The Family Allowances Act 1945 marked the first scheme of allowances to benefit *all* families with two or more children irrespective of the employment status of either mother or father and without proof of need or evidence of contributions" (Land, 1985, p 9). Frank Field stated, "It was a half-nurtured measure, but it nevertheless brought about a most profound change in fiscal and social policy. The living standards of children were to some extent to be decided upon by the nation as a whole, and were not any longer to be determined solely by the capriciousness of the market" (Field, 1996a). Professor Ruth Lister, a former director of the Child Poverty Action Group, recorded that the Act "represented a key building block in the post-war welfare state. It marked a recognition for the first time that the direct costs of children were the responsibility of the wider society as well as of individual parents" (Lister, 1999, interview with author). It is true that politicians have not always looked with affection at the national cost of family allowances. It is true that the financial levels of the allowances have not always kept pace with inflation, but they have survived and much credit must go to the Child Poverty Action Group for its part in maintaining them. The 1945 Act meant that mothers received, via the Post Office, an income of their own. Although, the amounts awarded by no means abolished poverty, they did remove the terrible destitution of the pre-war years which had driven some families to the Poor Law. Today, family allowances, now called child benefit and now applicable to the first child as well, continue as a source of money to all families with children and as an essential source to low-income families. Moreover, they are a popular source because entitlement requires no means test and carries no stigma. Most mothers and children are unaware of this, but there is a direct line between the money in their pockets and Eleanor Rathbone.

Deprived children

Much of this book is about people who championed the well-being of children separated from their own parents and often placed in the care of public bodies. So why start with Eleanor Rathbone? A major reason why parents are unable to cope with their children has been poverty. In pre-war Britain, hundreds of thousands of parents could not provide financially for their offspring and were forced to part with them to public bodies. The effect of poverty on parents was to undermine their health to the extent that they could not cope. The introduction of family allowances enabled far more families to stay together. Of course, the allowances were never sufficient and, in the 1960s, another champion, Peter Townsend, was among those who 'rediscovered' poverty and identified it as a continuing factor which undermined family unity. Nonetheless, in the years following the Second World War, family allowances were a major source of material help to low-income families.

But there is another link between deprived children and Eleanor Rathbone. As will be explained, Children's Departments were created in 1948 and required skilled staff. Few universities had trained child welfare workers, but one such university was Liverpool. Eleanor, along with Elizabeth Macadam and others from the Victoria Women's Settlement had, as Margaret Simey recorded:

> ... laid the foundations for courses of training which eventually formed the nucleus of the University School of Social Science, almost the first in the country. Eleanor played an important part in this, undertaking the lectures on local government and raising most of the necessary funds. Her subsequent long association with the School covered the emergence of the new breed of professional social workers. (Simey, 1974, p 14)

Not least, Eleanor always stood for the value of individuals. She sometimes spoke about social classes but she made it clear that classes were made up of unique individuals. She further insisted that every individual had an equal claim on society and also that every individual should be so raised that they were prepared to contribute to society. In the years just before and immediately after her death, other women, and some men, were applying such a principle to deprived children. Foremost was Marjory Allen.

TWO

Marjory Allen, 1897-1976

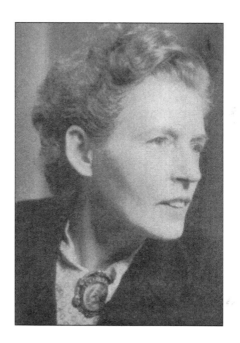

Photograph of Marjory Allen,
from *Memoirs of an uneducated Lady*
(Thames and Hudson, 1975)

As Chapter One describes, Eleanor Rathbone was instrumental in the establishment of family allowances, which eventually benefited all children in the United Kingdom. Marjory Allen, on the other hand, became known for her concern with the substantial minority of children who were separated from their own parents.

Eleanor Rathbone was born into wealth and what is often called 'the establishment'. She went to Oxford, had the money and the time to devote herself to social causes, and had the connections to ensure election as an MP. She did not marry, resisting social pressure to rely on an emotional relationship with a man. By contrast, Marjory Allen (née Gill) had a less privileged and more unusual background and enjoyed a lasting marriage. Both made significant contributions to major pieces of child care legislation in the 1940s.

Marjory was born on 10 May 1897. Her parents were educated, cultured people but with a strong sense of independence that made them the 'hippies' of their day. Her mother, Sala Gill, literally threw away her corsets when she threw herself into the movement for women's rights. Her father, Georgie Gill, was a rate collector for the Kent Waterworks Company who organised his colleagues into a guild in order to negotiate with their employers. One outcome was improved pension rights for the collectors, which Georgie promptly benefited from by taking early retirement. The Gills then raised their five children on this modest pension, which was supplemented by growing their own vegetables and fruit.

Unusually for the time, Sala and Georgie did not send their children to Sunday School. In fact they did not bother too much about sending Marjory to school, claiming that they could educate her at home. They were both artistic, and Georgie's cousin was Eric Gill, the well-known sculptor. On hearing about a new progressive and mixed boarding school called Bedales, Marjory's parents sent her there, at the age of 13.

Bedales

Bedales, which included a number of children from radical parents, was a culture shock for a young girl who had never even turned on an electric light. However, she soon proved that she was no pushover by tackling a female bully. Paradoxically, the young woman who was to be an ardent pacifist made her mark in a fight.

Bedales did not compel pupils to attend classes. Nonetheless, Marjory developed interests in book-binding, music and gardening. She learnt to be at ease in the company of boys and recalled that, in the early years of the First World War, one of her boyfriends, by then a fighter pilot, flew low enough over the school so as to drop her a love letter. Within a week he had been killed. The war horrified Marjory; she rebelled against the jingoism that others called patriotism, and became a life-long pacifist.

Marjory Gill never took an examination at Bedales. She later acknowledged her debt to the school by writing, in her autobiography written with the assistance of Mary Nicholson,

> I am glad I was not at a school where education was something of a hurdle race.... I had learnt that the happiness of achievement, so precious to children, is not found exclusively in academic or worldly success. This thought has guided me in my attempts to help children, intellectual or non-intellectual, physically handicapped or physically robust. For all

children, life should be, as it was for me, a continuous celebration, free from the pressures which can do irreparable damage to their self-esteem. (Allen and Nicholson, 1975, p 49)

Gardens and love

On leaving school in her late teens without any qualifications, Marjory was not sure what to do. She knew that she would not settle for being 'just' a wife and mother. She had heard that a well-known gardener, Edwin Beckett, was having difficulties in recruiting male staff because of the war. Beckett offered to take her on as a 'pot-boy' at ten shillings a week. She received no formal training but picked up a great deal of practical gardening knowledge. After a year, Marjory became confident enough to apply for the Diploma in Horticulture course at the University College of Reading. She was accepted despite her lack of qualifications. She then received a form to gain entrance to the hall of residence; under the section headed 'Religion', she wrote 'none'. The college wrote back to say this was not good enough and, if uncertain, she should write in 'Church of England'. Marjory refused. Weeks passed until the authorities gave in. Marjory wrote:

> ... the fierce and dictatorial warden of St Andrew's Hall never forgave me. Throughout my two years' residence I was almost always in her black books. I don't think she ever knew that I organised midnight excursions to bathe naked in the Thames but she obviously thought me capable of organising any crime. I got no credit from her for introducing lacrosse to the university, or for rowing stroke in the first women's university eight. (Allen and Nicholson, 1975, p 55)

Marjory had little spare cash but her charm ensured that she enjoyed an active social life. On one occasion, a boyfriend lent her his motorbike. Having never ridden one before, she roared away until, in Guildford, she realised that she did not know how to apply the brakes. Ignoring a policeman's signal to stop, she crashed. Two men stopped their car to assist her. One, a coffee planter on leave in Britain, became another romantic attachment and introduced her to the nightclubs of London. She also attracted attention from some of the college staff, and one of the lecturers promised her academic success if she would 'cooperate' with him. Marjory declined and in 1920 succeeded in gaining the Diploma on merit.

On leaving Reading, Marjory was invited back to Bedales to design a new garden. The result was so good that she began to win commissions. Her career seemed set. She was a founder member of the Institute of Landscape Architects and later earned some fame as the creator of the roof garden at Selfridges and the balcony garden at the BBC. Before these successes arrived, she had married Clifford Allen.

Clifford Allen was born in 1889 to middle-class parents. He was educated at private schools, the University of Bristol and Peterhouse College at the University of Cambridge. At Peterhouse, he rejected his parents' Christianity and became a socialist. He soon gained a reputation as a fervent speaker, attacked the institutions of the House of Lords and the monarchy, and helped to establish the University Socialist Federation. During the First World War, he founded the Non-Conscription Fellowship which recruited hundreds of members. However, it was immensely unpopular at a time when thousands of young soldiers were dying for their country. Brought before a tribunal, Allen argued that socialists believed in 'the brotherhood of man' and so could not take up arms against others. He was sentenced to hard labour in prison which he bravely endured, despite terrible conditions and a poor diet: he lost the use of one lung and nearly died; his health was ruined.

Released after the war, Allen found himself a Labour hero. He identified with, and became treasurer of, the Independent Labour Party, which was one of the more radical elements in the federation which made up the Labour Party. He seemed assured of a safe seat in the House of Commons and would probably have been selected to stand for the Gorbals constituency in Glasgow. Unfortunately, his lung condition worsened and he was forced to withdraw.

In 1921, Allen was recuperating in Italy. Marjory was also there, having sold her violin in order to spend some time with her artist brother, Colin. On one outing, Colin recognised some English friends, and in their party was Clifford Allen. Marjory later recalled that "He was tall and very thin, with a gaunt, handsome face" and she was immediately attracted to "this poetic, romantic person" who shared a flat with Bertrand Russell (Allen and Nicholson, 1975, p 62). Allen was used to female admirers but had never committed himself to any of them. His biographer, Arthur Marwick, explains that now Allen had fallen in love with a woman who was not only beautiful, but who possessed an independence of spirit and what Allen called "her goodness" (Marwick, 1964, p 7).

Once back in Britain, Marjory moved in with Clifford Allen. However, in the 1920s, it was not conventional for unmarried partners to live together openly and even Marjory's parents did not approve. Neither Clifford nor Marjory cared much about convention, but they did marry in December 1921, at Chelsea Registry Office. He was 32, she was 24. In September 1922, their only child, Polly, was born. Marjory wrote that they were then visited by Bertrand Russell, who "looked down at Polly and said, 'She will undoubtedly be a social worker', implying that this was the lowest form of human endeavour" (Allen and Nicholson, 1975, p 76). It would have amazed both Marjory Allen and Bertrand Russell to know that, years later, she was to contribute to the founding of Children's Departments which multiplied the number of social workers.

The Allens moved into their own specially built cottage in 1924. To her parents' distress, Polly suffered a brain haemorrhage which impaired her speech and sight. Fortunately, an outstanding surgeon enabled Polly to eventually make a full recovery. The stay in the new cottage was not to last. One of Clifford's rich, female admirers was in pursuit of him and bought land next to the Allens' as a prelude to moving there. Although Marjory was broadminded, she was unable to tolerate this. In 1928, they moved to Hurtwood in Surrey, where they built Hurtwood House.

With Clifford not in a permanent job, and Marjory not earning large amounts, how the Allens could afford a large house, gardener and housekeeper seemed to be a mystery. It was later revealed that Clifford was an expert player on the Stock Exchange. Strange contradictions began to emerge about Clifford Allen. He was a radical socialist who condemned the capitalist system, while simultaneously enjoying the money markets. He was a fine writer who attacked the desperate poverty and inequalities in Britain, while simultaneously adopting a lifestyle of affluence and seeking the company of the privileged.

Meanwhile, Marjory's career was blossoming. She won more commissions to design town gardens, including one from H.G. Wells. Her successes led to her writing a weekly 'Country Diary' for *The Manchester Guardian* which provided a regular income. Later, in 1936, she was made chairperson of the Coronation Planting Committee which initiated permanent schemes to mark the coronation of Edward VIII. The following year she became one of the first people to give a talk on television. She was on a programme which included two platinum-blonde contortionists, a Breton onion seller – complete with onions – and a champion female accordion player. The studio was hot, packed with the many attendants of King Boris of Bulgaria, who was in the audience. As Marjory opened her mouth to commence her talk, so the air was rent by the accordion as the champion player fainted and sprawled on her instrument.

Lord and Lady

Marjory and Clifford were determined that, despite frequent illnesses, Polly would have a relaxed and happy childhood. Clifford loved playing with and reading to her. Marjory joined with some neighbours to form a cooperative to run a nursery school under the leadership of Janet Jewson, a Froebel-trained teacher whose methods impressed Marjory and stimulated her interest in nursery education. Polly stayed at the school well beyond nursery age, and eventually followed in her mother's footsteps by boarding at Bedales.

Marjory's concern for nursery education led her to join the Nursery School Association in 1933. Later, she was commissioned to make a garden for a roof top nursery school in a new block of flats built for the St Pancras House Improvement Society. While doing this, she was introduced to adventure playgrounds, of which more will be written later. Almost without knowing it, the planner of gardens was being drawn into the world of children, and today she is remembered more for her contribution to this cause, than for her achievements in gardening.

During these years, the Labour Party twice held political power, although on both occasions its leader, Ramsay MacDonald, led governments which did not hold an overall majority of seats in the Commons. The second Labour government started in 1929, when Britain was entering a serious economic depression. MacDonald's economic approach was so cautious, and akin to that of the Conservatives, that it brought criticisms from sections of the Labour movement, especially the Independent Labour Party. Clifford Allen, however, strove to unite all elements under MacDonald's leadership. By 1931, 2.5 million people were unemployed. In order to obtain loans from abroad, MacDonald and his colleagues agreed to cut public expenditure. The Cabinet was divided and the government resigned (Holman, 1990, ch 7). To general amazement, MacDonald then stayed on as Prime Minister of a national government. As most Labour MPs refused to back him, it was essentially a Conservative administration. When MacDonald called a general election in 1931, during which he condemned most socialists as wasteful spenders, Clifford Allen campaigned on behalf of MacDonald. In the election, Labour was reduced to 46 seats, for which many blamed 'the traitor' MacDonald. To cap it all, Allen, despite his previous views on the House of Lords, accepted MacDonald's offer to be a peer. Allen's defence was that in the Lords he could help to save the Labour Party by calling on socialists to follow MacDonald. Former colleagues and friends poured scorn on him. Marjory Allen – now Lady

Allen of Hurtwood – cared little about titles but she did care about her husband and was prepared to accept his explanations.

By the mid-1930s, another world war seemed a probability. Clifford Allen had previously campaigned for peace, but now favoured the use of force against the aggressors. He refused to join the Peace Pledge Union in which members pledged not to fight in the next war. His apparent change of principle "was condemned by some old friends and colleagues" but his argument was that pacifism could not defeat fascism (Allen and Nicholson, 1975, p 136). Marjory remained a pacifist and admitted she could give only "unsatisfactory answers" to Clifford's new position (Allen and Nicholson, 1975, p 138). But she was fully at one with his tireless efforts to secure the release of a prisoner in Germany – Hans Litten, partly Jewish by birth, who had acted as defence counsel for several communists. He had been arrested and the attempts to secure his release failed; Litten was later found hanged in prison. Meanwhile Clifford Allen's health deterioated and he died in a sanatorium in Switzerland in March 1939.

The Second World War (1939-45)

In 1939, Marjory Allen was a widow with her only child still at boarding school. She was only 42 and a titled Lady with many political connections. She wanted to do more with her life, and the events of the war were to bring her the opportunity to do so.

As soon as the war began in September 1939, the government set in motion a large-scale evacuation of children and young mothers from urban areas to places which were considered safe from bombing. Chapter One explained how the evacuation made the poverty of many working-class children more public. Marjory Allen wrote that the evacuation "showed me the work I wanted to do. As a total pacifist I could take no part in the war effort, but I could help the children" (Allen and Nicholson, 1975, p 150).

Most evacuee children were placed with households, sometimes called foster homes. Young mothers with small children were also billeted with families. Marjorie wrote:

> They were placed in lodgings where the problems of two women in one kitchen were never solved. Often enough they had nowhere to cook or do their washing, and they were sometimes expected to be out of the

house from early morning until blackout time. Then their lives consisted of wandering up and down the road, dragging their little children with them wherever they went. Lonely and overstrained, it is small wonder that many of them lost heart. Small wonder, too, that the under-fives often suffered from lack of suitable food, lack of quiet rest and a lack of opportunity for exploratory play. They urgently needed a place of their own, where friction was reduced to a minimum, where prohibitions were not all-important and where they could make a noise and exercise their natural curiosity without troubling their mothers, foster mothers or landladies. In short, they needed nursery centres. (Allen and Nicholson, 1975, pp 151-2)

By this time, Marjory was on the executive of the Nursery Schools Association and began to campaign for nursery provision for evacuees. In June 1940, the government issued a circular urging local authorities to set up nursery centres and guaranteeing to cover the costs involved. The local authorities were slow to respond because they were having to cope with a multitude of difficulties created by the influx of evacuees, and because there was a shortage of staff, suitable space and equipment.

The Nursery Schools Association quickly set up short training courses which qualified those who completed them to work as nursery assistants. The next step was to second a staff member to work in Guildford, which held many evacuees, where Marjory demonstrated that space could be found for small groups. Meanwhile Marjory contacted the British War Relief Society of America with whom, no doubt, the title Lady Allen of Hurtwood was well received. The society agreed to make a grant for 10 regional organisers who not only initiated new centres, but made use of prefabricated buildings to put them in. Marjory travelled the country, in dirty, crowded and unlit trains, to make speeches and seek support. She persuaded Herbert Morrison, the Home Secretary, to visit the centres in Guildford.

In 1942, now chairperson of the Association, Marjory was worried that not enough equipment could be found for the growing number of centres. In London, she observed the huge amount of debris from bombed buildings. Again, she went to Herbert Morrison, who was won over by her, and agreed that civil defence workers could separate useable wood from the other debris. She then organised a large number of craftsmen, often Quakers and other conscientious objectors, to construct toys, chairs, tables and other equipment. In 1943, an exhibition of the goods was opened by Morrison who was by now almost eating out of her hand.

The membership of the Nursery Schools Association trebled to over 9,000. The war had facilitated the creation of a better nursery service for children.

J. Arthur Rank agreed to make a film to show how a good nursery school should work. It was launched in November 1943 with the Duchess of Kent as guest of honour. George Bernard Shaw agreed to attend, apparently because he had heard of the Duchess' beauty. On entering the room, he mistook Marjory for the Duchess and fell on his knees before her. The film brought J. Arthur Rank and Marjory into contact and he saw her as the person to help him. He had started Saturday morning films for the war-time children but the films were so boring that the kids often went wild. He invited Marjory to chair a body to advise on suitable films, which she did by asking the children what they liked and wanted to see.

Marjory did not limit herself to nursery centres for evacuees. The number of day nurseries multiplied under the auspices of the Ministry of Health, but Marjory disliked their domination by health personnel, matrons, nurses and by doctors who "tended to regard children only as bundles of tummies and throats that were breeding grounds for germs" (Allen and Nicholson, 1975, p 166). She criticised the unstimulating environments in some day nurseries, and stated outright that children under the age of two should be with their mothers. She also said that those aged two to five years required a happiness which "comes from creative play and constructive occupation" (Allen and Nicholson, 1975, p 167).

Her pleas and criticisms had little effect on day nurseries, however. She therefore deemed it even more essential that there should be more nursery schools, that they should be an integral part of education policy, and should be forced on local authorities as a mandatory and not a permissive service. With a new education Act in the offing, the Nursery Schools Association sent several deputations to R.A. Butler, the president of the Board of Education. She recorded, "To our great satisfaction the 1944 Education Act established that nursery schools and classes were a part of primary education, and a duty was laid on local authorities to provide nursery education for children under five" (Allen and Nicholson, 1975, p 170). Unfortunately, the implementation of this provision was postponed by government after government and Marjory never saw its fulfilment.

Deprived children

Although Marjory was disappointed that the legislation regarding nursery education was put aside, she was soon in the thick of another campaign which was to result in effective legislation. Marjory later wrote, "My own efforts during the war to extend an understanding of nursery education soon led me, by chance, to stumble on another subject which kept me occupied for several years" (Allen and Nicholson, 1975, p 170). She was referring to what she initially called "homeless children" and later "children deprived of a normal home life". It is significant that Marjory Allen, for all her involvement with young people, had never before encountered such children. The reason was that for years they had not been in the public eye and therefore not on the political agenda.

Before describing Marjory's next achievements, something must be said about the history of services for deprived children. In Western society, church bodies have long provided for children who do not have adults to look after them. As the power of the 'mediaeval' church declined, so other organisations were forced to do more. The 1601 Poor Law Relief Act instructed local parishes to accept responsibility for destitute children. Voluntary bodies also grew, reaching a peak in the 19th century with such famous child care societies as Dr Barnardo's Homes, the National Children's Homes and Orphanage and the Waifs and Strays Society. At the time of its founder's death in 1905, Barnardo's was looking after 11,277 children. The Poor Law, by the end of the 19th century, was responsible for the care of 58,000 children in workhouses, children's homes and residential schools, plus a further 8,000 boarded-out with foster parents.

During the early decades of the 20th century, national concern for deprived children declined. There were no national figures of the stature of Dr Barnardo to keep them in the public eye. The voluntary societies looked after over a thousand children's homes, yet a number were in financial difficulties and much of their drive had been lost.

The Poor Law was criticised for its large and regimented children's institutions. In the 1930s, its functions were handed over to local authorities who ran the institutions through what were usually called Public Assistance Departments; but to working-class people it was still the same Poor Law. By now, local authority Education Departments were displaying more interest in the social, physical and medical needs of pupils. London County Council authorised the setting up of children's care committees which used trained volunteers to visit families whose problems were adversely affecting their children's education. The seminal 1933 Children and Young Person's Act, with similar legislation for Scotland in 1937, widened the definition of children who could be brought before the courts as in need of care and protection. When the courts placed fit person orders on such children, it was local authority Education Departments who took on the responsibility for them. Consequently, the departments expanded their residential and fostering services, although these were always seen as having less priority than the departments' main function of running schools. Within the Home Office, a handful of liberal inspectors, influenced by the growing discipline of psychology and books like Cyril Burt's *The young delinquent* (Burt, 1925), were struggling against the tide to reform approved schools. Some child psychiatrists and social workers were developing methods of treating emotionally deprived children in child guidance clinics. But their efforts were small against the vast and almost stagnant system of child care.

Despite modest advances, there seemed little prospect of large-scale improvements at the end of the 1930s. The majority of children whose parents could not look after them were still in residential institutions, many of which were very big and staffed by untrained personnel. The administration of child care was fragmented between a host of different central government, local government and voluntary agencies. The deficiencies of child care were not a matter of political concern. Even if they had been, the prospects of reform were slim given that the government of the day was committed to retrenchment, not increased expenditure. And then came the Second World War.

Evacuation led to the large-scale removal of children from their own homes, and their placement with other people. It put separated children back on the public agenda. The children's responses to separation in terms of bed-wetting, aggressive behaviour and emotional unhappiness were taken seriously. Academics looked into how foster parents should be selected. Opinions were voiced that deprived children deserved a better service. Someone with vision, drive and political clout to draw these strands together was needed, and that person was Marjory Allen.

Marjory records that in her frequent visits to schools, "I gradually became aware of groups of children who looked different from the others. They were fat, flabby and listless, and wore heavy, ill-fitting clothes and boots so clumsy that they could only shuffle along. They looked overfed and unhappy, and never seemed to join others in the playground" (Allen and Nicholson, 1975, pp 170-1). Marjory was informed that they were from children's homes. She admitted that she knew little about such children but was determined to improve her knowledge. Her initial efforts to see inside the homes were rebuffed. Local officials did not cooperate and she observed, "I failed at first to find anyone actively interested" (Allen and Nicholson, 1975, p 171). Not easily deterred, she knocked at the door of a children's home which had been evacuated to a large Victorian house at a seaside town. The nurses, who ran the home for 50 boys, greeted her kindly and showed her around. The staff considered that the children were lucky to have such a good home, with food and shelter. However, Marjory saw it through different eyes. For instance, she disliked the playroom, which was, she stated,

> ... large, chilly, unhomely and sparsely furnished. The boys were standing around, unoccupied. They showed little curiosity and were very shy when I spoke to them. I asked where they kept their toys and was taken to look at a cupboard. Except for a few broken toys, the shelves were bare.

> My guide took me to the dormitories, which had drab walls and identical dull grey bedcovers. There were no personal treasures to be seen, no pictures on the walls, no sign that anyone had tried to create a warm, cherishing atmosphere. (Allen and Nicholson, 1975, p 171)

She was informed that persistent bed-wetters were caned in the chapel.

This visit acted like a social accelerator for Marjory. She sought out further homes. She went to grouped cottage homes where the organisers proudly claimed that each cottage reconstituted the family. Marjory was not convinced – some cottages were restricted to children of a certain age and gender, and some had huge iron gates to keep the children away from the outside community.

Marjory was pleased to find some local authority homes which were located in ordinary, terraced houses so that the children were not obviously marked out as different from other children, where they went to local schools and played in the street. She also saw statutory homes which were large and impersonal. But her anger was particularly directed at voluntary bodies who cast the stigma of 'charity children' on the residents of their homes. In one county town, she observed 'charity' girls walking in crocodile formation and wearing identical long, dark cloaks. Locals referred to them as 'the bastards'.

Marjory's next step was to find out who was responsible for the statutory homes and who inspected the voluntary ones. She discovered that, at central government level, children's homes were run by the Ministry of Pensions, by all three branches of the armed services and by the Ministry of Health, while the Home Office was responsible for approved schools. At local authority level, Public Assistance Departments and Education Departments had numerous residential institutions. Responsibility for inspecting voluntary homes was spread among various central government departments. It was, as she put it, "a super-colossal" muddle.

As she pursued her new interest, Marjory met with other concerned people. Psychiatrists John Bowlby and Donald Winnicott were writing about the adverse effects on children of badly run institutions. Magistrates Basil Henriques and John Watson and the well-known academic and former welfare worker, Mary Stocks, were also asking questions about the treatment of children. Marjory made friends with Leila Rendel, the director of the progressive Caldecott Community, who had long taught that children could benefit from residential homes where skilled staff treated them as individuals. These experts knew more about the psychology of deprived children than Marjory, they had much more experience of seeing them in the courts and in residential settings. Marjory's genius, however, was that of getting things done.

Her letters to government departments asking for the numbers of children in public and voluntary care, how they were treated, what action was taken on inspectors' reports and so on were being met with bland, evasive responses. In consultation with her new colleagues, she decided to bring the matter to the public by a letter to *The Times*. This letter, published on 15 July 1944, has a place in child care history and deserves to be given here in full:

> Sir, – Thoughtful consideration is being given to many fundamental problems, but in reconstruction plans one section of the community has, so far, been entirely forgotten.
>
> I write of those children who because of their family misfortunes, find themselves under the Guardianship of a Government department or one of the many charitable organisations. The public are, for the most part, unaware that many thousands of these children are being brought up under repressive conditions that are generations out of date and are unworthy of our traditional care for children. Many who are orphaned, destitute, or neglected still live under the chilly stigma of 'charity'; too often they form groups isolated from the main stream of life and education, and few of them know the comfort and security of individual affection. A letter does not allow space for detailed evidence.
>
> In many 'Homes', both charitable and public, the willing staff are, for the most part, overworked, underpaid, and untrained; indeed, there is no recognised system of training. Inspection, for

which the Ministry of Health, the Home Office, or the Board of Education may be nominally responsible is totally inadequate, and few standards are established or expected. Because no one Government department is fully responsible, the problem is the more difficult to tackle.

A public inquiry, with full Government support, is urgently needed to explore this largely uncivilised territory. Its mandate should be to ascertain whether the public and charitable organisations are, in fact, enabling these children to lead full and happy lives and to make recommendations how the community can compensate them for the family life they have lost. In particular, the inquiry should investigate what arrangements can be made (by regional reception centres or in other ways) for the careful consideration of the individual children before they are finally placed with foster-parents or otherwise provided for; how the use of large residential homes can be avoided; how staff can be appropriately trained and ensured adequate salaries and suitable conditions of work, and how central administrative responsibility can best be secured so that standards can be set and can be maintained by adequate inspection.

The social upheaval caused by the war has not only increased this army of unhappy children, but presents the opportunity for transforming their conditions. The Education Bill and the White Paper on the Health Services have alike ignored the problem and the opportunity.

Yours sincerely,
Marjory Allen of Hurtwood

Marjory Allen was anxious that her letter might have little impact. People were still preoccupied with the war as the allies fought their way through France. Pilotless planes, known as 'doodlebugs', were dropping on London and another evacuation of children was underway. Yet she need not have worried. Sir William Haley, himself a later editor of *The Times*, wrote about her letter:

> The response was staggering. Day after day and week after week the letters poured in. Many came from leaders in social work and others who had also first-hand experience. Even after the normal correspondence had been closed, *The Times* had to publish no fewer than

six round-ups of further letters. (cited in Allen and Nicholson, 1975, p 180)

Marjory followed up the correspondence by getting MPs to put questions to ministers about the numbers of children in voluntary homes, about which homes were inspected and about how often homes were visited. The responses were hardly satisfactory. In response to a question about what was done with the inspectors' reports, the Minister of Health simply replied that the reports were filed. However, it was established that homes which had endowments, and which did not ask the public for money, were not inspected at all. Finally, 158 MPs signed a request for an inquiry. On 7 December 1944, Herbert Morrison announced that an inquiry would be made.

In private, Morrison told Marjory that she had overstated her case (Allen and Nicholson, 1975, p 184). He took no action to name the members of the inquiry. Marjory decided that another push was needed and set about writing a pamphlet which drew on the many letters, often from staff and former children of children's homes. She worked so amazingly swiftly that it appeared in February 1945.

Whose children? is a classic campaigning pamphlet of just 32 pages (Allen, 1945). Marjory starts by defining the meaning of deprived children. This definition includes those children "with an unsettled home background or no home background; orphaned and illegitimate children; those with chronically ill parents; the destitute; children on probation; and others who have been compulsorily withdrawn from their parents" (Allen, 1945, pp 2-3). Her objective was to speed the government inquiry, and her main criticisms of the child care system were four-fold.

First, she reported, children's homes were too institutionalised, too much organised for the sake of the system and too little for the sake of the individual child. Marjory acknowledged that the physical care of children was usually satisfactory, although some provided the children with a poor diet. She was, however, much more concerned about emotional care. She wrote of five-year-olds in homes with no toys and, worse, no attachment to an adult. Staff were often so obsessed with physical cleanliness that children had to spend much of their time cleaning and polishing. She doubted if children residing in large institutions which were isolated from the outside world could be prepared for the time when they had to move into the outside community.

Second, children were not only unready to leave care, they also received little help when they did so. Girls were often put into domestic service where they felt lonely and neglected. Boys were often directed into the armed forces. Both types of jobs meant that they did not get accommodation of their own. Worse, in Marjory's view, was the practice of some charities of retaining girls as cheap domestic labour. Other young people were sent out with little help in finding jobs and with no one to whom they could turn.

Third, Marjory criticised the institutions' staffing. She wrote, "The staffing of the present Institutions and Homes seems to be the worst single factor and the most crucial" (Allen, 1945, p 24). Staff were often overworked. In one case, one man and three students were in charge of 250 boys; this was exceptional but it was usual for a housemother to have the sole responsibility for 10-14 children. Not surprisingly, staff were often so overworked that they had "little time to give individual and personal attention to the children" (Allen, 1945, p 25). Moreover, they suffered from a lack of training, low wages and poor living conditions.

Fourth, Marjory attacked administrative confusion. She pointed out that the child care system was fragmented between so many different agencies that resources were wasted and bureaucracy multiplied. She headed one section of the pamphlet, "Whose concern are these children?" (Allen, 1945, p 26). There was no one body, no one ministry, no one department responsible for deprived children. They were all within agencies where priority was given to other duties. Consequently, the nation lacked child care leadership.

Following her strident analysis, Marjory asserted that deprived children had to be part "of the main stream of life" (Allen, 1945, p 32). To this end, she made a number of specific recommendations:

- An extension of fostering. She argued that a foster home was much more akin to a normal family than a children's home. However, she acknowledged that the fostering service needed improvements in order to recruit better foster parents, to pay them higher allowances, and to supervise them more closely.
- More humane children's homes which would entail small homes replacing the larger institutions. As a model, Marjory praised the hostels set up within the evacuation schemes for children who did not fit into foster homes. She wrote, "In these small Hostels, under the oversight and protection of trained psychiatrists or social workers, children have found that individual study, care and affection which alone can help them to recover from the loss of their homes or from damage inflicted by bad homes" (Allen, 1945, p 19).

- With regard to staffing, she declared, "The most urgent reform is to establish a nationally recognised system of training and to ensure adequate salaries, conditions of work and pensions" (Allen, 1945, p 26).
- The establishment of a reliable system of inspecting children's homes.
- She wanted, for deprived children, "the unification of administrative responsibility, both central and local"(Allen, 1945, p 32).
- She ended the pamphlet by writing, "The public has been too content to accept without question ... the work that has been done in their name and with their money. We must see that the public eye, the most efficient inspector, should be kept constantly vigilant and alert" (Allen, 1945, p 32).

Whose children? received enormous publicity. Over 59 newspapers and magazines featured it. Some reactions were negative, even hostile. Two members of the London County Council and some senior officials of large voluntary societies implied that Marjory Allen was condemning all children's homes and all residential staff. The criticism was unjustified for, in the pamphlet, she had pointed out that good practice existed and, indeed, had urged that the government inquiry should draw attention to the "many good and happy Homes ... as an inspiration and example to others" (Allen, 1945, p 2). It was even implied that she was making money out of the campaign. The charge was quite false: in fact, she had put her own money into it. In public, Marjory gave the impression of being thick-skinned yet these attacks hurt her. In her autobiography she reveals "[I] wondered if I was tough enough for this kind of battle" (Allen and Nicholson, 1975, p 191). Fortunately she possessed a wide range of friends who encouraged her to persist. She makes particular mention of Bob Trevelyan, a classical scholar and poet, who had been a friend of Clifford's and whose photograph appears in the autobiography. She wrote that he was the one "above all, [who] knew how to give me solace" (Allen and Nicholson, 1975, p 191). Marjory and her colleagues must also have been heartened by the overwhelming number of responses to *Whose children?* which were positive and which put added pressure on the government to start its promised inquiry.

Other events were also highlighting the need for action. In January 1945, a foster child, Dennis O'Neill, was so badly treated by his foster parents on an isolated farm in Shropshire that he died. Herbert Morrison appointed Sir James Monckton to examine the tragedy and his report quickly attributed the blame to inadequate supervision by untrained staff within a framework of fragmented services. Even before appointing Monckton, however, and soon after the publication of *Whose children?*, the Home Secretary, on 8 March 1945, named the members of two committees "To enquire into existing methods of providing for children who, from loss of parents or from any other cause whatsoever, are deprived of a normal home life with their own parents or relatives; and to consider what further measures should be taken to ensure that these children are brought up under conditions best calculated to compensate them for the lack of parental care". Myra Curtis, principal of Newham College, Cambridge, was appointed chair of the body to report on England and Wales, while the senior Scottish judge, James Clyde – who was soon to become Lord Advocate – headed up the committee for Scotland.

Noticeably, Marjory Allen was not included, although the press had taken her appointment for granted. Marjory confronted Herbert Morrison about her omission. He replied that she had already made up her mind and could not be objective about voluntary societies. Some consolation came from the fact that Myra Curtis obviously valued Marjory's contribution and invited her not only to give written and oral evidence to the committee, but also to provide a list of points which members should consider when visiting children's homes.

The Clyde and Curtis Reports appeared in 1946. They were presented to the Labour government which had swept to power and replaced the war-time coalition government in 1945. The Clyde Report, *Report of the committee on homeless children* (Scottish Home Department, 1946), argued strongly for an emphasis on fostering, which was the closest approximation to family life, whereby the child "secures the necessary opportunity to build up its own personality and equip itself for the transition to independence and self-reliance" (Scottish Home Department, 1946, para 45). It argued that an expansion of fostering and improvements to children's homes would not come about in a fragmented service and it called for a new local authority children's committee with sole responsibility for deprived children, staffed by trained officials. The Clyde Report was a mere 36 pages. John Murphy, in his history of Scottish services, points out that "Neither the Scottish public nor press was clamouring for changes", which he attributes to the fact that Scotland lacked a Dennis O'Neill and a Lady Allen (Murphy, 1992, p 26).

The Curtis Report, *The report of the care of children committee* (Home Office et al, 1946), five times longer than its Scottish counterpart, was, as it stated, "the first enquiry in this country directed specifically to the care of children deprived of a normal home life" (Home Office et al, 1946, para 3). It included 'delinquent' as well as 'deprived' children in its brief and calculated that their numbers were 124,900. It made a detailed investigation of residential establishments and concluded that many were too large, too isolated, and too institutionalised. Like the Clyde Report, it argued that children fared better in foster homes. Its masterly analysis ended with 62 recommendations, of which the following were the most significant:

- The order of preference for care provision for children unable to live with relatives is adoption (although this was applicable to only a few children), followed by fostering, then residential care.
- Responsibility should rest with one local authority committee with its own department, to be overseen by one central government ministry.
- The children's committee should employ its own executive officer (later called the children's officer).
- Training should be introduced for all staff.
- Voluntary societies should have a better system of inspection.

The reports were milestones in the history of child care in Britain. No previous studies had so clearly identified the failings of the current system of child care and made such pertinent recommendations. No previous writings had so powerfully made the case for child care agencies which put children first and which emphasised the right of every deprived child to personal care and individual attention. However, Marjory did have some reservations and, in a letter to *The Times* on 16 October 1946, argued that children resident in voluntary homes should still be in the care of local authorities. But she was probably pleased on two scores. First, many of the recommendations were in line with those she made in *Whose children?*. Second, the public, press and parliamentary responses to them were almost wholly positive and the government made it clear that it would prepare legislation.

The Children Act became law on 5 July 1948. It stipulated that local authorities be given a duty to receive into their care children under the age of 17 whose parents or guardians were unable to provide for them, and whose welfare required the intervention of the local authority. It established local authority children's committees which were also to take over responsibility for children committed to local authorities by the courts, for the protection of private foster children, for the supervision of certain adoption placements and for the inspection of voluntary homes. The committees' responsibilities were to be executed by a single department, the Children's Department. The Home Office was designated as the responsible central government department. The Act decreed that local authorities had a duty to board-out (foster) children in their care and, when this was not practicable, to maintain them in residential homes. It established an Advisory Council on Child Care to advise the government on the promotion of training.

The 1948 Children Act has received little attention from political historians. Morgan, in his *The people's peace: British history 1945-1989*, praises the welfare legislation of the post-war Labour government but does not mention the Children Act (Morgan, 1990). Even more surprisingly, the Prime Minister, Clement Attlee, who was once a social worker, gives it no attention at all in his autobiography (Attlee, 1954). Yet it was a profound, humane and effective statute. It meant that no more destitute children would fall within the provisions of the Poor Law. It meant that the importance of deprived children was recognised by the establishment of local authority committees – and their departments, the Children's Departments – which concentrated just on them. Jean Heywood, the notable children's historian, wrote that the Act contained a clause "perhaps unmatched for its humanity in all our legislation" (Heywood, 1959, p 158). She was referring to the general duty placed on local authorities, "Where a child is in the care of a local authority it shall be the duty of that authority to exercise their powers with respect to him so as to further his best interests, and to afford him opportunity for the proper development of his character and abilities" (1948 Children Act, Section 12). As Heywood points out, this duty replaced the Poor Law legislation, which was abolished in 1948, that the authorities should "set to work or put out as apprentices all children whose parents are not, in the opinion of the Council, able to keep them" (Heywood, 1959, p 158).

The Children Act was not, as some writers imply, due just to Marjory Allen. Even before the war, criticisms were being made of children's services and suggestions made for improvements. The Second World War itself stimulated huge changes in Britain, not least of which was a change in public attitudes which welcomed the establishment of a welfare state. The evacuation opened a door which put deprived children on to the public stage and drew in practitioners, academics, politicians and foster parents, who then displayed their concern for such children. Nonetheless, it was Marjory who engaged the interest of a large audience and many then considered the deficiencies of the system of child care for the first time. It was Marjory who brought people and ideas together and forced politicians into action.

After the 1948 Children Act

The passing of the Children Act was probably the high point of Marjory Allen's public life. From 1950-51, she served on the Advisory Council on Child Care. She maintained her interest in child care and often spoke at conferences. Brian Roycroft later became a well-known children's officer and director of a social services department. In the late 1950s, he was just starting as a child care officer. In an interview with me, he recalled that he went to a conference where he met Marjory Allen. He said:

> She questioned me very intently about how relevant my training had been and then asked what I was doing about the fostering of older children. About a year later, I was invited with four others to talk with her about how the Children Act was working out. The discussion went on all afternoon with the main subject being prevention. I think she was collecting material for the lobby to bring in what was eventually the 1963 Children and Young Persons Act. At the end, she asked me to stay behind and asked me why more men were going into child care. Then she probed again about fostering and asked me whether, once a child had been through several foster homes, it was best to stop. I said there was a time when it was best for a child to settle into the security of a children's home. She had a sharp, decisive mind and sought out great detail such as what did the children look like, what did they wear. I felt she was seeing them as people, not just cases.

> When I became children's officer of Gateshead in 1963, she wrote me an encouraging letter. And again when I moved to Newcastle. She was an encourager. (Roycroft, 1999, interview with author)

Marjory maintained her interest in nursery education and was prominent in the World Council for Childhood Education. In 1949, she was appointed as the Social Welfare Liaison Officer to the United Nations International Children's Emergency Fund (UNICEF). Based in Paris, she was soon immersed in programmes to alleviate the sufferings of children in a Europe which was still recovering from war.

Marjory returned to Britain in 1951. It was a bleak period for her. Bob Trevelyan died. She could no longer afford to maintain Hurtwood House so she and Polly moved into a cottage in Sussex, where she gained much pleasure from cultivating its garden. But she still wanted to be active and now had the opportunity to develop her interest in adventure playgrounds. She defined an adventure playground as "a playground where children are provided with miscellaneous equipment, often waste material, from which they may contrive their own amusement" (Allen and Nicholson, 1975, p 233). She joined the committee of Clydesdale Road Playground in North Kensington. In 1953, she wrote another influential pamphlet for the National Playing Fields Association called *Adventure playgrounds* (Allen, 1953). It contributed to the interest in and the growth of adventure playgrounds throughout Britain.

Age did not lessen Marjory's attractiveness and, in 1954, Herbert Morrison asked her to marry him. She records that her decision to decline was a difficult one, for they had become close friends. Morrison was aggrieved and she never saw him again.

Her involvement in the adventure playground movement was expressed in the part she played in setting up the London Adventure Playground Association in 1962, whose chairperson she remained for 10 years. At the age of 68, she undertook an exhaustive and exhausting lecture tour in the USA. Three years afterwards she published a book entitled *Planning for play* which proved to be popular (Allen, 1968). Then she met a friend of Polly's living in a London basement flat with three children, one of whom was severely disabled. Marjory believed that disabled children also needed playgrounds tailored to their requirements, so she set about promoting them, and there followed another pamphlet, *Adventure playgrounds for handicapped children*, published by the Handicapped Adventure Playground Association (Allen, 1973).

Marjory moved to a terraced house in London with a small garden, near Polly who had a job in the city. With her friend Mary Nicholson, she set about writing her autobiography. She sensed that her life was drawing to a close and her last published words were "The work I have chosen to do is never finished" (Allen and Nicholson, 1975, p 260). She was talking about her work with children. She died on 11 April, 1976 at the age of 78.

An uneducated Lady

Marjory Allen was an unlikely children's champion. Other figures in this book displayed a concern in their twenties for deprived or poor children. They were soon active in social reform movements or child care agencies. When in her twenties Marjory was much more interested in gardens and landscapes. She was, however, a woman of deep feelings and principles. Her parents' influence and the influence of her school made her tolerant of others and in favour of liberal, even permissive, educational regimes. She was a pacifist from her teens until her death, and she was in sympathy with the Labour movement. She was most comfortable with those who held radical views. No doubt her political awareness was sharpened by her relationship with Clifford, but it is difficult to identify exactly just when her interest in child care reached the point when she decided to become a public campaigner. I have suggested that the turning point probably came with motherhood, when she became involved in nursery education for her own daughter, and wanted this kind of experience to be available to other children. Oddly enough, the woman who hated war found that the Second World War was a kind of social springboard that threw her into campaigning for and demonstrating the value of nursery centres for evacuees. Her activities made her a well-known figure and she used this to her advantage.

She was a latecomer to the world of deprived children and this may explain some of her limitations. Much of her analysis was not original. Criticisms of the institutional nature of children's homes were being made long before the war. In her biography of John Bowlby, Suzan Van Dijken notes how he and other child psychiatrists had observed both the ill-effects of separating children from their mothers at an early age, and the limitations of residential homes and schools whose staff gave little time and individual attention to their charges (Van Dijken, 1998, ch 3). Not least, official committees had pleaded, in vain, for improved salaries for social workers. It must also be added that she was not well read in child care. She never mentions the influential children's care committees of London City Council. She mostly ignores the growing child guidance clinics and the theories and treatment approaches they were developing. She was apparently ignorant of a number of writings about good residential child care. Despite her protestations, there is some substance to the charge that she was prejudiced against the voluntary child care sector. She did make justifiable criticisms but she did not always present a balanced picture. In *Whose children?* she vehemently attacked the poor after-care provided by voluntary societies. But there were some voluntary homes whose after-care was much more advanced. Marjory would have preferred all deprived and separated children to be 'wards of the state'. To have done so certainly would have saved some children from unacceptable standards of care in some voluntary homes. But it would also have thrown out much of the positive experience and good practice that others offered. Marjory also wrote little about the destructive influences of poverty on children's lives.

These limitations do not serve to detract from Marjory Allen, however. If anything they enhance her. She was the foremost child care figure in the1940s despite the lack of a background steeped in child care agencies, child care psychology and child care practice. Why was she so influential?

She was very persuasive. Her attractive personality and looks were supplemented by what Barbara Kahan called, in an interview with the author, "a certain vitality" (Kahan, 1999, interview with author). These qualities made her not a formidable figure but a very appealing and engaging one. No doubt her marriage to Clifford Allen and her title gave her access to powerful people. She then used these contacts to persuade officials, committee members and politicians, to her point of view.

She had passion. She opened *Whose children?* by claiming that deprived children needed another Charles Dickens, one who was all heart as well as intellect, one who would tread "the road of fearless exposure" (Allen, 1945, p 1). She herself was a kind of female Dickens. Although she did not write lengthy novels, she wrote short, terse, moving pamphlets which vividly exposed the plight of needy children. Her suggestions may not all have been original, but she grasped the cause and was passionate about it. Perhaps her passion was all the greater because awareness of the sufferings of deprived children was new to her. Unlike the liberal Home Office officials, who perceived the drawbacks of institutional regimes, she was prepared to seek publicity in the popular press. Unlike some academics, she was prepared to take on the bureaucracy who wanted to uphold the system that suited them. She was deeply angered by the treatment of deprived children. As she wrote in the foreword to *Whose children?*, "I am not alone in being ashamed and indignant at many of the things that can happen today in this world of children. But to make men desire better things requires that we should first reach the human heart: and that is the purpose of this pamphlet" (Allen, 1945, p 2).

Marjory rapidly grasped the essentials of the child care system and saw its strengths and weaknesses. If her analysis was not new, some of her proposals definitely were ahead of contemporary thought. If, as John Bowlby and others were asserting, children fared best with their own parents, then she wanted the new Children's Departments to support parents in order to prevent children having to go into care. The 1948 Children Act did not go that far – it placed a duty on local authorities to try to return children to their families but did not empower them to prevent their admission in the first place. Again, she was radical, in the sense that she wanted services for unmarried mothers so that they did not necessarily have to place their children for adoption or into public care. Not least, she wanted to know "that [children] have the right to appeal to a public body, such as the suggested National Children's Trustee if they are in difficulty or in need of help of any kind" (Allen, 1945, p 20). Only in the 1990s did the issue of the rights of deprived children become a major issue. In 1939, although Marjory's knowledge about deprived children was much less than that of the child care experts, by 1949, her vision was ahead of them.

Finally, she was influential because she was a skilled organiser. She marshalled the limited forces of the Nursery Schools Association to maximise its pressure on government. She cooperated with scores of people concerned about deprived children, she organised them to speak, write and exert pressure. She was prepared to take the lead herself, although she was not, by nature, a dominating person. Barbara Kahan (the subject of the next chapter) recalled of Marjory:

> She described to me in detail how she organised *The Times* correspondence. She said if you want to get something done you have to keep at it for months. She described how she had sent letters to the three government ministries every month for a year asking what they were going to do. She never got proper answers. Once her letter appeared in *The Times*, she developed a rota with other people to keep letters going in to the paper. The editor kept trying to close it down but had to re-open it. I thought she was marvellous. (Kahan, 1999, interview with author)

In 1939, the plight of materially and emotionally impoverished children rarely featured in the mass media. War, evacuations and the re-emergence of the Labour Party as a political force, created a climate in which change was accelerated. In 1945, the Family Allowances Act moderated, but by no means abolished, child poverty. Much of the credit went to Eleanor Rathbone who had striven for decades for reform. In 1948, the Children Act established the first local authority service just for children separated from their own parents. Much of the credit went to Marjory Allen, who had striven for just a few years. Whatever the reasons, whoever the champions, the fact was that Britain now had a two-fold service for children. First, there was a central government ministry organising universal financial provision for all children (except, to begin with, for the first born child) which was of particular help to poor children. The question then became whether the provision would survive and whether its value would be

THREE

Barbara Kahan, 1920-2000

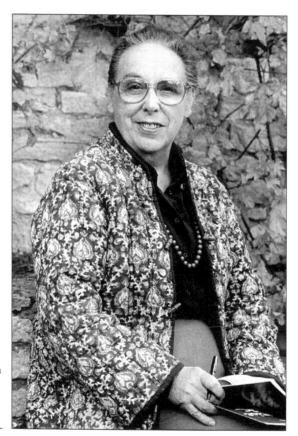

Photograph of Barbara
Kahan, kindly supplied
and published by
permission of
Community Care

In his book, *Child welfare in England 1872-1989,* Harry Hendrick makes
no mention of Barbara Kahan (née Langridge) (Hendrick, 1993). Yet
anyone involved in the day-to-day practice of children's services since
1948 knows the name of Barbara Kahan well. Indeed, they probably
know it better than that of any other figure in child care. As a local
authority practitioner, senior civil servant, writer and campaigner, she was

always to the forefront. As there is no other full account of her life, it is timely to record and review her contribution.

Early life

Barbara Langridge was born in Horsted Keynes, Sussex. A family life rooted in the railways – both her grandfather and father were station masters – is not an obvious preparation for a life devoted to professional child care. But it was a family which immersed her in intellectual, religious, social and political stimuli. Her grandfather read constantly to the young Barbara from books ranging from fairy stories to the *Pilgrim's progress* to the Bible. Ill-health, particularly asthma, prevented her from attending school until she was over six years of age, but by this time she was already an avid reader. Her grandparents and parents alike were fully involved in a Methodist chapel. Barbara was then drawn into a culture in which the belief in and the practice of serving others played a major part. Barbara's mother was a very intelligent woman who had won a scholarship to a grammar school where she thrived, but when she was 16, her family moved and the scholarship was non-transferable. By way of compensation she devoted much of her life to helping others and was determined, as Barbara put it in an interview with me, "that my brother and myself should have a clear message about how to live" (Kahan, 1999, interview with author). At the age of eight, Barbara was delivering food, which her mother had cooked, to people living in poverty. At that time, her parents were strong supporters of the Labour Party. It was thus instilled into her not only that she personally should help individuals, but also that social improvements could be advanced by political action.

Barbara soon had her chance to help others at the grammar school to which she had won a scholarship. During the 1930s, many Jewish people were attempting to leave Germany and the school's headmistress told the assembly about one girl who needed a home in Britain. Barbara promptly suggested to her mother that they could take in the girl, and her mother quickly agreed. The girl moved in and never saw her own parents again, but remained a member of the Langridge family, with Barbara always referring to her as her 'foster sister'.

Barbara won a state scholarship to Cambridge University in 1939. University was a turning-point for her. She helped to re-start the university Labour Club and worked for Richard Acland's egalitarian Commonwealth Party. She studied English Literature and people expected that she would become a schoolteacher. Instead, on graduation, Barbara moved to the

London School of Economics, which was in war-time residence at Cambridge, where she obtained a distinction in every paper on the social studies course.

In 1943, inspired by a lecture from an inspector, Barbara applied for, and obtained, a post as a government inspector of factories in the Midlands. As an inspector, her eyes were opened to the poor working conditions of many employees. As a civil servant, she soon grasped the virtues of careful record keeping and administration. But the job never satisfied her. From newspapers she learnt about the campaign of Lady Allen of Hurtwood to improve the lives of deprived children. She read and wept over the Curtis Report. She was determined to work among such children and applied for the newly created post of children's officer for Dudley.

Dudley Children's Department

Barbara was called for an interview at the small borough of Dudley. She recalled:

> There were five other applicants, all at least ten years older than me. The interviewing panel was enormous, including one member who fell asleep. I had no experience except for youth club work in my spare time and, to my amazement, they offered me the job. I was very young and they could not appoint me until confirmation was received from the Home Office. (Kahan, 1999, interview with author)

Barbara started in July 1948 as a new officer in a new department responsible for implementing the new 1948 Children Act. Sitting in the one room allocated to her, she was surrounded by files sent over from the Public Assistance Department. Within half an hour, a parent arrived wanting her child taken into care. Not knowing what to do, Barbara ran for advice to the chairman of the children's committee who, fortunately, lived close by and he explained the procedure for receiving a child into the care of the local authority. After six weeks, she received permission to employ a 17-year-old secretary. For months, Barbara was visiting and interviewing families single-handedly. Exhausted, she contracted double pneumonia but was soon back at the job she had grown to love. A chief clerk and two child care officers were acquired and they too were prepared to work 12-14 hours a day. Much time was spent trying to find accommodation for the children and, on more than one occasion, Barbara and her colleagues took children into their own homes.

The difficulty in finding accommodation was partly due to the fact that Dudley had no residential establishments of its own and relied heavily on placing children in a village of cottage homes run by Wolverhampton. Barbara frequently visited the Dudley children who lived there and took them to the zoo and on other outings. Before long the children's officer of Wolverhampton asked for the outings to be stopped as it upset the children placed by other authorities who were not taken on such outings. Barbara was furious. She ensured that children in the care of Dudley received as personal a service as possible. Letters and cards were sent to them by staff. Individual Christmas and birthday presents were bought, wrapped and sent. Outings were arranged and visits made so that they had opportunities to talk personally to their child care officers. Barbara then persuaded Dudley to open its own children's home.

During two busy years at Dudley, the young children's officer seized on three aspects of child care which were later to be closely associated with her name. One was preventative work, that is, efforts to stop children being needlessly removed from their parents and received into public care. In legal terms, the 1948 Children Act stated that children should be returned to their families if desirable but did not sanction expenditure on prevention. Nonetheless, the more radical children's officers did start to experiment, and Barbara was one of them. Her department moved into a house with offices on the ground floor and accommodation for a family upstairs. The teenage children of this family and other young people started to join in the staff lunches where they soon relaxed and were able to communicate. Barbara felt that a closeness to families was a key to prevention. A second aspect to prevention was intensive work. In one case, the National Society for the Prevention of Cruelty to Children (NSPCC) obtained a court order to remove two children when their mother had a third child in conditions of squalor. The children's father was partially sighted and the mother had had a deprived childhood. A dedicated child care officer, however, recognised that, with help, the parents could probably care for their children themselves. Barbara explained:

> While the mother was in hospital and two children in care, the father and department staff worked together to clean, decorate and make ready their home for a possible return. Second hand furniture was obtained, rent arrears put on hold, and at the court hearing the magistrates were asked to put the children back at home under supervision from the Children's Department. It was agreed that initially daily budgeting would take place and daily help of many kinds be ensured. The case

appeared in the national press under the heading 'The Smiths get a housekeeper' but the outcome was such that, a year later, health visitors were able to say that the family's care of the children was as good as other families in the area. (Kahan, 1999, interview with author)

Barbara was convinced that many more children could remain at home. Her enthusiasm and thinking was, as Terry Philpot later pointed out, all the more remarkable at a time "when the professional axiom was that the sooner a child was separated from his 'bad' family background the better: then the slate could be wiped clean – even if it meant life in an institution" (Philpot, 1977).

The third aspect of child care closely associated with Barbara's name concerned the treatment of young offenders. She recalled, "I went to the juvenile court and discovered that children were being sent to approved schools for the most trivial offences, like stealing a few sticks of rhubarb from a front garden" (Kahan, 1999, interview with author). In one case, a white girl aged 16 fell in love with a black boy aged 17. The girl's father was so angry that he brought her to court as 'beyond control' and she was committed to a girls' approved school. Barbara accompanied the girl and expressed her concern to maintain contact with the girl and said she would help wherever possible. The school's headmistress made it clear that she was in charge and wanted a clean break between the local authority care service and the approved school and coldly brushed aside Barbara's offers of assistance. The result was that Barbara could not maintain a close relationship with the girl but she then determined to do something about approved schools.

Dudley was responsible for 72 children in care plus supervision of private fosterings and those placed for adoption. Barbara was interested in every one of these children and wrote one of the first reports about the work of a Children's Department (Kahan, 1949). It made an impression on Kenneth Brill, the then children's officer in Devon. Years later and towards the end of his life, Brill undertook a PhD about the history of Children's Departments, in which he highlights the importance of the Dudley Report (Brill, 1991).

First, Brill pointed to the intensive yet friendly nature of the work with families. Previously, such families had tended to come under the auspices of Public Assistance Departments, whose officials kept a distance, emphasising regulations and conditions. The Dudley child care officers were different, and Brill praised the friendly relationships between child care officers and families.

Second, Brill highlighted the Report's concern to improve and extend the fostering of children. The Curtis Report and the 1948 Children Act recommended fostering in place of institutional care. Yet, in the early years of the Children's Departments, some were so overwhelmed by the numerous applications for care that they could give little time to expanding and improving fostering. Not so in Dudley, however. At a time when 'physically' and 'mentally handicapped' children (to employ the terms then in use) were often not considered suitable for foster homes, Brill highlighted "the successful fostering of a severely handicapped three year old boy who wept at the sight of strangers, suffered from night terrors and had a distended abdomen and legs too weak to carry him" (Brill, 1991, p 76).

Third, Brill noted the establishment in Dudley of a system of weekly time sheets completed by child care officers. These sheets made it possible to analyse how staff spent their time and the kind of cases with which they coped. Brill observed that they also revealed "the stresses imposed on staff during the early years" (Brill, 1991, p 74).

But Brill was not the only one to notice the Dudley Report; it was widely circulated and read. Barbara received an appreciative letter from Eileen (later Dame) Younghusband, the leading social work figure of the time. Barbara's name was noted. Moreover, the positive response to the Report probably confirmed Barbara in her own belief that she had something to contribute to child care. She applied for the post of children's officer in the much larger authority of Oxfordshire.

Oxfordshire Children's Department

In January 1951, again in the face of older and more experienced candidates, Barbara got the job as children's officer for Oxfordshire. The contrast with Dudley could hardly have been greater. Dudley was a small borough, with under a hundred children in care, dominated by councillors who lived close to the council offices. Oxfordshire was a large county, with nearly 400 children in care, which was run mainly by Conservatives and Independents including some powerful aristocrats. Barbara explained:

> The chair of the county council was an earl who nominated all the chairs of committees. In a deeply Tory county, the Labour party appeared to be allowed anything that was not considered important and that included the children's committee. Its chairman was a railway signalman and I was told to go to the signal box if I wanted to talk with him. (Kahan, 1999, interview with author)

Barbara soon felt that not all the committee members were sympathetic. Some of the Labour members held the view, "These kids have had a rough time but so did I and I managed" (Kahan, 1999a, interview). The Conservative attitude was reflected in the councillor who objected to children in children's homes having treats such as ice cream. Despite the size of the county, the Children's Department had a small staff establishment made up of a deputy children's officer and just three child care officers. With regard to residential provision, it had three old-fashioned establishments on one campus, a long-stay children's home, a remand home and two nurseries. Moreover, there had been little time to set up the department's administrative procedures and framework. Hardly a promising start, yet Barbara was always to be associated with Oxfordshire and remained its children's officer until Children's Departments were abolished. She made a decision – as she put it, "I felt I had to make a choice between being a nice girl or a battle-axe: a nice girl they would pat on the head and ignore; a battle-axe would give them a bit of trouble and they would have to think twice before they dismissed what she said. I chose the latter. What else could I have done if I wanted to achieve anything?" (Kahan, 1999, interview).

The new children's officer soon put the department on a sound administrative footing. Her drive and efficiency won over many of the committee members, who agreed with her request for more child care officers who were professionally qualified. As in Dudley, she was deeply concerned about the standards of residential care. Homes were made more homely while staff benefited from regular consultations. Child care officers were required to visit children regularly and to share reports with residential staff. Perhaps Barbara's greatest achievement in residential care at this time was to recruit trained staff. Qualified residential workers were hard to find and even harder to keep. In Oxfordshire the percentage went up to over 50% compared with just 15% for the rest of the country.

No matter how good the standards of care away from home, Barbara remained convinced that most children fared best if they stayed with their own families. As a member of the Association of Children's Officers, she had put forward her views on prevention which, by the mid-1950s, were gaining some ground. The foremost child psychiatrist, John Bowlby, wrote in his famous *Child care and the growth of love*: "... the basic method of preventing a child from suffering maternal deprivation must be to ensure that he receives nurture within his own family" (Bowlby, 1953, p 99). Barbara therefore encouraged health visitors, teachers and the NSPCC to refer needy children to the Children's Department before their difficulties became so great that removal could not be avoided. Coordination and cooperation with other officials was important, but Barbara knew that the essential ingredient was the quality of the relationship between child care officers and families. In 1952, she appointed to Oxfordshire a staff member with experience in a Family Service Unit. He was given a small caseload of what were then called 'problem families' and became a familiar figure as he drove around in an old van in which he transported clothes, furniture and people. He won the trust of suspicious and previously rejected families, and succeeded in improving their circumstances so that many child placements into care were prevented. The achievement was all the more remarkable in that – in these post-war years of chronic housing shortages – some lived in deplorable conditions including an encampment of old huts. Barbara persuaded the children's committee to help fund a voluntary organisation to place a social worker on this site doing preventive work. Barbara was never one to keep her distance, so she visited the huts and, at Christmas, organised the celebrations at which she played the piano.

Prevention was advocated because it was regarded as in the best interests of the emotional health of children. Policy makers added their approval because it was cheaper than taking children into care. Oddly enough, however, Barbara was also pursuing a strategy that actually ended up taking more children into care. With no holds barred, she pursued her conviction that approved schools were damaging to children. She spent time explaining to magistrates what the Children's Department could offer as an alternative to approved schools. Child care officers developed skills in writing reports on offenders for courts. The strategy was successful. Approved school committals in Oxfordshire fell dramatically so that during a period of six years only one child from Oxfordshire was resident in such a school, and he had been committed by a court outside of the county. Between 1953-65, 88 young offenders were committed to the county's care and of these only 16 appeared before the courts again. And the magistrates were still happy to leave the 16 with the Children's Department and not send them to approved schools (Packman, 1975). Meanwhile, the little known 1952 Children and Young Persons (Amendment) Act placed on local authorities a duty to investigate any information suggesting that a child was in need of care and protection whether or not the apparent neglect was 'wilful'. This authorised progressive Children's Departments to intervene before children came to court and, hopefully, to divert them away from public care.

Jean Packman, now a leading child care researcher but formerly a child care officer and later deputy children's officer in Oxfordshire, argues that one of Barbara's greatest achievements was her recognition "that delinquents were not a separate breed of children all of whom needed to be locked up" (Packman, 1999, interview with author). In the 1950s, this view was counter to the strongly entrenched belief that deprived children needed care while 'delinquents' needed punishment. Barbara first fought her case in Oxfordshire in order to change local practice and later went nation wide in order to change legislation. But it was a pitched battle with her opponents, locally and nationally, who argued that she was 'soft' on crime, that she was more concerned about the young 'thugs' than their victims. In Oxfordshire, the other main criticism levelled against this young, radical children's officer was that her policies increased county expenditure. As the courts committed more offenders to the care of the local authority so the costs fell on the local authority rather than on approved schools, which were mainly financed by central government. Barbara convinced most of the children's committee that the expenditure was justified but the finance and general purposes committee and some senior officials were alarmed. They persuaded the Home Office Child Care Inspectorate to investigate. It reported that the Children's Department was providing an effective service. Further visits from the organisation and methods officer and from an investigator sent by the finance and general purposes committee came to nothing. Barbara's response was always to provide all the information they wanted, to invite them into the Children's Department and to take them to see the work that was being done. Such was the quality of the work and the strength of Barbara's arguments that they often became allies. Barbara was still in charge of one of the smallest departments within Oxfordshire; she was its only female chief officer and she had taken on and not succumbed to the arguments of more senior officials that she was spending too much money. And she did not do so by becoming a 'battle-axe'. She won by her powers of persuasion, by her marshalling of figures to support her claim that prevention was cheaper than custodial care, by her passion, by her resilience and, at times, by her charm.

In Dudley, Barbara had attempted to improve standards of foster care. In Oxfordshire, she encouraged child care officers to check every prospective placement against the prediction table found in Roy Parker's *Decision in child care* (Parker, 1966). Oxfordshire supervised far more adoption placements than Dudley, and she soon became concerned about adoption standards. She encouraged pregnant, unmarried women to turn to the child care officers for advice and help rather than make haphazard adoption placements through the private market. Later, a regional group was established which drew together other nearby Children's Departments, voluntary adoption societies and moral welfare workers. Members pooled information and set down guidelines concerning the selection of adopters, the manner of placements and the regularity of supervisory visits to the children once with the prospective adopters. They were establishing standards that were later to become widespread and to be enshrined in legislation.

It was an adoption case which confirmed Barbara's growing belief that non-accidental injury (or child abuse) was more widespread than commonly thought. A paediatrician from a hospital – close to but not in Oxfordshire – rang to discuss a child who had been placed for adoption and whom he had admitted into the hospital with a fractured skull. The records showed that a previous adopted child of the couple had also suffered a similar injury. The adoptive parents were middle class and well-esteemed in the local community. Barbara went straight to the police and a senior officer subsequently rang to say that he was satisfied that the mother had dropped the baby after tripping over the doorstep. Barbara was not so easily satisfied and approached the voluntary society which had made the placement. The society was resistant but Barbara insisted that the child's interests and not the feelings and needs of the adoptive parents had to come first. Eventually, the child was removed by the society. Two years later, the husband came to see Barbara to seek placement of another child for adoption. In the very difficult circumstances, the best that Barbara could do was to make it clear that not only would the department not place a child with the couple, but, if application was made to a court in the county concerning another placement, the court would be told the full facts as known (Kahan, 1999, interview with author).

Oxfordshire Children's Department was one of the first to emphasise the need to respond urgently and positively to the problems of child neglect and physical cruelty, although in the early years of the implementation of the 1948 Children Act this tended to be seen as the traditional task of the NSPCC. Barbara pointed out that, in Oxfordshire, "The development of preventive work was an integral part of a strategy which ranged from prevention through protection, rehabilitation and ongoing support after return home if that was possible" (Kahan, 1999, interview). However, she acknowledged that her department, like others, was not fully alerted to the dangers of sexual abuse as it was understood in later years. Years after she left her post, she was visited by two sisters who had been in the care of Oxfordshire. One revealed that she had been distressed by the sexual advances of her foster father and that it took a long time before her child care officer would take her complaints seriously.

The other sister suffered similar advances in another foster home which were so serious that she attempted suicide as a means of escaping from the placement. Later, Barbara said that she and others were not aware of the scale of sexual abuse and consequently were not adequately alerted to what some children were trying to tell them.

During the 1960s, Barbara was a prominent member of the Association of Children's Officers; in 1964 she served as its president. Along with a few other key children's officers – she especially praises Kenneth Brill of Devon, Ian Brown of Manchester, Bill Freeman of Sheffield and Sylvia Watson of Hertfordshire – she liaised with local and central government figures and became a well-known public speaker. Therefore, she knew many Children's Departments and was in a good position to evaluate them as a whole. She acknowledged that some of the departments were too small, did not attract qualified staff and did not promote high child care standards. Overall, however, she was certain that the departments had a beneficial effect. She identified three main achievements. First, she argued that the Children's Departments "turned a minimalist Public Assistance service into a much more personalised and child-centred service" (Kahan, 1999, interview). Children in care were treated more like children in their own homes, particularly with regard to standards of food, clothing and pocket money. Barbara was delighted that the old practice, whereby children were seen as a readily available supply of domestic servants and labourers for local gentry and farmers and as entrants to the armed forces, was replaced by the concept that children's abilities should be developed to the full. Child care officers in many, but certainly not all, Children's Departments were encouraged to befriend the children, to take them out, and to understand their needs.

It was these officers whom Barbara identified as the second great achievement. The new service succeeded in recruiting a highly motivated staff. She stated, "The child care officers were well educated, they knew the law, they were systematic. Many were attracted into the work just because it was with children. The task of trying to compensate children for what they had lost fitted well with a feminine approach to life for many of the early child care officers were women" (Kahan, 1999, interview). In a later publication, she explained that, within the Children's Departments, the professional occupation of child care developed more quickly than other branches of social work. It thus contributed to social work, establishing itself "as a parallel not subsidiary professional service with health and education" (Kahan, 1970, p 59).

Third, she considered that the Children's Departments took a promotional view of their work. Local authority departments were often reactive, waiting to see what duties central government would place on them and then waiting for individuals to walk through their doors. Children's Departments, by contrast, were often proactive. Their staff often encouraged not discouraged people to use them. Departments like Oxfordshire wanted the police, teachers, and health officials to refer their clients to them. In turn, the Association of Children's Officers and Association of Child Care Officers lobbied politicians for legislation which placed further responsibilities on the Children's Departments. Far from living up to the media image of a bunch of hesitant 'fuddy-duddies', the staff of the Children's Departments frequently conveyed a sense of enthusiasm and mission, which was to seek change.

One personal event of great importance to Barbara occurred during her years in Oxfordshire. In 1951, she met Dr Vladimir Kahan. Vladimir was born in London in 1907, his father having come to Britain from Latvia, his mother from Poland. After medical training, Vladimir married and joined his father as a general practitioner in East London. With the advent of the Second World War, he served abroad as a psychiatrist in the Royal Army Medical Corps in Iraq, Persia and India. He returned to London where his father had died, the medical practice was destroyed, and his marriage suffering from his long absence. He had served with Dr John Bowlby and their friendship reinforced his desire to specialise in child psychiatry. After further training, in 1947 he was appointed director of the Oxford and Oxfordshire Child Guidance Services. He possessed a tremendous rapport with children of all ages and later, as a consultant with the NHS, developed a special interest in autistic children.

Barbara and Vladimir were married in 1955. The marriage was a huge success. She admired his broad intellectual capacities and learned from his medical and psychiatric knowledge. He admired her drive, determination and enthusiasm. They shared a love for music, art and for giving parties for councillors, officials, child care officers, students and anyone with a commitment to children. Jean Packman, who knew them both well, amusingly explained that they were like Picasso portraits, larger than life, "vivid, colourful and warm.... There was always liveliness, laughter and even the occasional rows were entertaining" (Packman, 1999, interview with author). Vladimir was not slow to express his feelings, including anger, and Jean Packman recalled "...Vladimir savagely berating an idea or a person in his soft, light, dry voice, while Barbara pleaded for moderation and compassion in her ringing, operatic tones" (Packman, 1999, interview). Barbara was at pains to explain that Vladimir had not changed her child care values and practices.

Rather he provided the reassurance and the knowledge base that she was on the right track. Vladimir also had the capacity to tease his wife gently, and to get her to laugh at her own foibles. Jean Packman said, "Vladimir was a tremendous influence. She was inspired by him. It was an idyllic relationship" (Packman, 1999, interview).

The Seebohm changes

By the late 1960s, Barbara Kahan was a national figure within child care circles. In articles, lectures and conferences she argued against the false distinction between 'deprived' and 'delinquent' children. She asserted that the troubles of both had their origins in malfunctioning families, adverse environments and deprivation, and that it was no answer to place them in approved schools which were linked with punishment and stigma. Her work attracted the interest of Alice Bacon MP, then Minister of State in the Home Office, who accepted an invitation to come to Oxfordshire in 1965 and to see for herself the work being done and the alternatives offered. The minister was positive about what she saw and made it clear that she accepted the argument that 'delinquent' children had to be treated within the context of their families and neighbourhoods. After much debate inside and outside of Parliament, the 1969 Children and Young Persons Act effectively ended the approved school system and emphasised a care rather than a punishment approach. However, it should be added that the Act was never fully implemented following a change of government and as a result of the reorganisation (to be discussed below), Children's Departments were absorbed into much larger services.

Meanwhile, even larger changes were on the cards. As Children's Departments expanded their preventative work and their involvement with offenders, so they appeared to be more like a family service than a children's service. The suggestion was put forward that a new family service should incorporate not just Children's Departments but parts of other local authority services which dealt with the family. Scotland was ahead of England and Wales in this regard and the 1968 Social Work (Scotland) Act amalgamated Children's Departments with other personal social services into social work departments as well as setting up Children's Hearings as a new way of dealing with young offenders. In 1965, in England and Wales, the government appointed Frederic Seebohm to chair a committee "to consider what changes are necessary to ensure an effective family service". Barbara was in favour of change and wrote much of the evidence submitted to the Seebohm Committee by the Association of Children's Officers. It acknowledged the case for a larger family service which would bring together duties currently fragmented between several departments. However, it wanted to exclude services for older people and disabled adults, along with mental health services and medical social work services in hospitals, at least until a later stage. It favoured a new family service, which would take over the duties of Children's Departments as well as day care, school welfare and young offenders.

In a collection of essays, published by the Fabian Society as *The fifth social service* (Townsend et al, 1970), Barbara wrote a more personal account. She reasoned that the expansion of Children's Departments into work with families and offenders meant that its staff were already becoming social workers rather than child care officers. They were then perceiving that the families' difficulties were often associated with "housing shortages, policies in allocating housing, social security limits and distribution and social attitudes to such minority groups as unmarried mothers" (Kahan, 1970, p 62). She concluded that a larger department was required both to encompass various types of family problems and also to be powerful enough to negotiate with other services – particularly those which controlled housing and social security – on behalf of the families. However, she did not want the new service to be too large and insisted that it should not be "a combined health and social work department" or that it should be headed by anyone "other than a fellow social work professional or a social work administrator with social work experience" (Kahan, 1970, p 64). She feared that any amalgamation with local health services would lead to former medical officers of health taking control, with social work being treated as inferior to health care.

Although Barbara wanted the new service to have a social work orientation, she pushed for a broad definition of social work which would include residential work and group work as well as casework with individuals. She added, in the Fabian pamphlet, that social work "is being pushed by events to make a decision as to whether it continues to be a way of helping people to sort out and put up with intolerable situations ... or whether, in addition to that, it must accept the role of a pressure group within society, commenting on intolerable situations and seeking to remedy them by means of national policy as well as individual supportive work" (Kahan, 1970, p 65). Barbara was thus an advocate of what later became known as 'radical' social work.

When the Seebohm Report finally appeared in 1968, it recommended a large, multi-tasked social services department (SSD). Although the department was larger than what she had wanted, the Report also contained two chapters which particularly appealed to Barbara Kahan. One was on prevention, in which it was argued that "An effective family service must be concerned with the prevention of social distress" (Home Office, Ministry of Education and Science, Ministry of Housing and Local Government and Ministry of Health, 1968, para 427). The other was on community in which the Seebohm Committee stated it wanted services accessible to all the community, with users participating in the running of services. These chapters were music to the ears of Barbara who longed for a service which would support families before difficulties escalated into problems, and which would be so widely used that it would not convey any stigma to users. She therefore became an enthusiastic campaigner for the implementation of the Seebohm Report.

In fact, legislation did come in 1970. It is ironic, perhaps, that Barbara Kahan, who was acknowledged as one of the foremost children's officers and who had built the Oxfordshire Children's Department into one which was admired throughout Britain, was also a leading player in the events which led to the 1970 Local Authority Social Services Act, which actually abolished the Children's Departments. The departments were amalgamated with welfare departments, mental health departments and sections of other educational, housing and health services into SSDs. In other words, the new local authority service was for adults as well as for children. The Act made no mention of prevention or community, but nonetheless, Barbara remained hopeful that a larger, more resourced, more politically powerful department would lead to a better deal for children and families.

At this time, the tireless Barbara was also fully absorbed in two other pieces of work. One involved a study group established by the Residential Child Care Association, the Association of Children's Officers and the Association of Child Care Officers which considered the role of residential child care. Largely written by Barbara and Geoffrey Banner, a residential worker who later became a director of a SSD, it was published in 1968 as *The residential task in child care*, although it was often known as the Castle Priory Report (Residential Child Care Association et al, 1968). It gave particular attention to the staffing needs of children's establishments and laid down a formula for calculating the numbers of staff needed in them. Two years later, the Home Office accepted its guidelines on staff ratios. The other piece of work was published in 1974 as the *Report of the committee on one-parent families*, known as the Finer Report (DHSS, 1974a). Barbara was a most active participant in this report, which argued forcefully for a guaranteed maintenance allowance, so that lone parents would not be forced into employment; for expanded day care for those who did wish to work; for improved housing, as well as many other recommendations. The immediate legislative impact of the report, to Barbara's disappointment, was slight. But it had established the economic and social difficulties of one-parent families while also showing that lone parents were not feckless, inadequate welfare dependants. Years later, the arguments bore fruit when lone parents were awarded extra financial benefits and governments began to develop a clear child care strategy.

The SSDs began to appoint directors in 1970. Barbara Kahan seemed to many to be the obvious choice as director of the Oxfordshire SSD. She had shown herself as a strong administrator and a leader who had won the loyalty of her staff. She had a national reputation as one of the leaders in social work. Yet, as one of her admirers, Jean Packman, pointed out, "Her convictions were so strong that she was bound to clash with some people. She can be alarming, she can be very fierce, people love her or hate her. So she made enemies" (Packman, 1999, interview with author). She also had a number of professional enemies among those who regretted the abolition of the approved schools. Certainly Barbara wanted the job, but the odds were stacked against her. She had won battles over money for the Children's Department and, in so doing, had left in Oxfordshire a residue of wounded and defeated enemies who did not want her to head the new department. Barbara revealed that, "The Clerk of the Council indicated that, while I was highly regarded, I spent too much money and was unlikely to be appointed" (Kahan, 1999, interview). After a long talk with Vladimir, she decided not to apply.

In late 1969, Barbara was urged by the then chief inspector to apply for the post of deputy chief inspector in the Home Office Children's Department. She was interviewed and accepted the post in January 1970. A year later, when that department was amalgamated with the Department of Health and Social Security (DHSS), Barbara became an assistant director in the Social Work Service. She served there initially with Joan Cooper and then William Utting. She was responsible for a development group, and for the nine regional groups of the Social Work Service (later called the Social Services Inspectorate), whose task was the inspection of services in SSDs and advising them on practice, legislation and government guidelines. At headquarters she was responsible for liaison with the NHS and the development of social work within the Health Advisory Service.

Barbara was not content to be a reactive civil servant and she particularly directed her enthusiasm into a development group to promote and evaluate new ideas and practice. It had a small budget and never more than five staff, but Barbara devised an approach which drew in many outsiders, usually people in middle management from various disciplines, who met and then re-met in seminars, spreading over a period of three years. The proceedings of one notable project undertaken in conjunction with the Welsh Office were published in 1977 as *Working together for children and their families*. Its focus was "the interface of concern and responsibility between personal social services and education for children with special problems and needs" (DHSS and the Welsh Office, 1977, p 4). An example given concerned children's truancy. It was explained that truancy might involve not only schools, but the SSDs, the health services, voluntary bodies, the police and the courts. The worry was that the fragmentation of services and differences in methods of treatment were not in the interests of the child. The project stemmed from Barbara's basic premise that solutions could not be imposed from above, but rather had to involve practitioners. Consequently, the participants included teachers, social workers, magistrates, probation officers, members of the police, nurses, education welfare officers, members of voluntary agencies, and local authority councillors. They were divided into groups, each with a separate task dealing with such topics as clarification of roles, the organisational basis of services, training, resources and communication. The outcomes were not revelations but they did enable participants to identify differences in values and procedures which hindered communication, and these findings led to a scheme for greater uniformity in record keeping, and a proposal for greater joint training for different occupations involved with children. Not least, the project brought together officials and representatives who had never before spent much time in each other's company.

A number of socially important issues were raised by the development group, such as child abuse, violence, standards of social work and, of course, residential care. Jean Packman and her partner, the academic, Bill Jordan, were invited to a series to improve services in one local authority. Jean recalled, "Barbara put her all into it. She was determined that standards would be raised. It was a very lively conference and succeeded in kick-starting changes in the services" (Packman, 1999, interview with author). Barbara's combination of 22 years' practical experience, her ability to conceptualise about policy matters and her great drive made her an ideal development person. She would not hear of an inspection approach which was negative and 'nit-picking'. She believed inspectors should be positive, encouraging and dynamic. Her one regret about these years was that residential care stagnated. She declared, "Nobody had the guts to replace approved schools with anything. There was a wholesale destruction of residential facilities which was a disaster" (Kahan, 1999, interview).

One reason why residential care was overlooked in these years was that little attention was given to the voices of the children who lived in care. This accusation could never be levelled at Barbara Kahan. As a children's officer she had insisted on communicating with children in the homes for which she was responsible. In 1969, she drew together 10 young adults who had grown up in the care of Oxfordshire Children's Department. They met together with Barbara and two colleagues over a period of a year and from the tape recordings of the discussions a book was produced, which was published as *Growing up in care* (Kahan, 1980). It was one of the first studies of the views of users of social services.

Some retirement!

In 1980, Barbara retired from the DHSS. She did not of course retire from social activity and she addressed numerous conferences, wrote many articles and took on private consultancies. Above all, she had the opportunity to pursue her concern for residential work. A number of social work notables, including the Reverend Nick Stacey (the director of Kent SSD), Godfrey Issacs (the chair of the well-known residential establishment, Peper Harow), Mary Joynson (the director of Barnardo's), and Janet Mattinson (an academic) had raised money – mainly from the Gatsby Foundation – for a project to improve the training of residential staff. The post of director of the Gatsby Project could have been designed for Barbara. Sadly, soon after she started, Vladimir was struck by an illness from which he died in February 1981. His death was a devastating blow for Barbara. She organised a memorial service at which she and friends met together to talk about Vladimir. Somehow she was able to carry on and, during a visit to the University of Victoria in Canada, she encountered its newly launched approach of distance learning for far-flung students. Barbara immediately perceived that this was a method that could be adapted to train far more residential staff in Britain. After long negotiations, she persuaded the Open University to organise, and the Department of Health to fund, such courses. They developed innovative and imaginative course books, supplemented by audio tapes and videos, which were both widely used and praised. The courses could be used by students in their own locations and work places with tuition from local Open University staff. They continue to this day, and the Open University and University of Victoria eventually awarded honorary doctorates to Barbara to mark her achievements in child care.

During 1983-90, Barbara also served as professional advisor to the House of Commons Select Committee on the Social Services. She thus influenced the seminal *Second report from the social services committee: Session 1983-84, Children in care* (House of Commons, 1984). Chaired by Renee Short MP, the report covered many topics but focused in particular on the prevention of children entering public care. This was timely, for prevention had passed out of fashion in social work. Instead, what was known as the 'permanency movement' had taken over, with emphasis on giving children permanent placements even if this meant cutting off their ties with their parents, siblings and their neighbourhoods. The report did not deny that the interests of some children were best served by permanent removal from their natural families, but it argued that the pendulum had swung too far and that the importance of children maintaining contacts with their relatives was being neglected. Therefore it called for a renewal of prevention:"... there is as yet regrettably little indication of any concerted strategy which could translate pious thought into action" (House of Commons, 1984, para 30). It urged local authorities to develop services – such as child minders and daily fostering – to enable more parents to cope with their own children. It wanted SSDs to appoint managers with special responsibility for rehabilitating children who were in care. It urged 48 legislative changes in order to protect natural parents from the over-zealous and hasty removal of their children:

> Not even the Seebohm Report had given prevention such priority. Moreover it was the first major official document to pose a serious challenge to the doctrine of permanency.... By identifying the features which impaired prevention and by stating quite specifically how it could be promoted, the Short Report made an important contribution to the case for prevention. (Holman, 1988, pp 91-2)

Barbara's involvement meant that she was simultaneously pursuing two of her great concerns: prevention and residential care.

Just as the Gatsby Project and Barbara's involvement with the Select Committee were coming to an end, so she was catapulted into another major child care arena. In 1990, she was about to leave for a well-deserved holiday when a telephone call from Staffordshire County Council invited her to join Allan Levy QC to conduct the Pindown Inquiry. Barbara postponed her holiday. 'Pindown' was the name given to an approach to control children in some of the residential establishments run by

Staffordshire SSD. It was alleged that the staff and the methods were repressive and cruel. Barbara cooperated well with Allan Levy QC who, she said, was "honest, committed to children and demanding to work for" (Kahan, 1999, interview). Over a six-month period, they often put in 12-14 hours a day as they interviewed 153 witnesses and studied 150,000 pages of evidence. Jean Packman said that Barbara excelled in making "sense out of messy situations" and that she showed a lawyer's capacity to ask searching questions and to sum up evidence (Packman, 1999, interview). Their findings, published in 1991 as *The Pindown experience and the protection of children*, demonstrated that senior staff had established an oppressive regime which controlled and punished children by keeping them in solitary confinement, depriving them of possessions, clothing and contact with others (Kahan and Levy, 1991).

But it was not enough for the report to uphold many of the allegations. It also had to ask how had the SSD allowed such a regime to be established? The authors identified the beginnings of the regime in the closing down of a number of children's homes in order to save money. This meant, for instance, that in one 15-bed home there were 28 young people. In order to cope with so many children, staff carried out harsh punishments which they later justified as a child care method which challenged children and made them confront their difficulties. Moreover, with a shortage of places for children, social workers had little choice but to send children to these homes despite any misgivings they may have had. The report showed that, in a large department, residential care had become buried beneath five layers of management, with the result that top officials and councillors were out of touch with reality. Indeed, the report strongly condemned the department for being unaware of what was going on over a period of nearly six years. Whatever the reason, the senior residential staff had been left untouched and therefore exercised considerable power, ran their own regime, threatened junior staff and ensured that children were unable to complain.

The report had an immediate and major impact. It was the main feature in all newspapers. The Department of Health immediately wrote to all local authorities requiring a report within one month as to whether any other homes followed similar regimes. Subsequently, Sir William Utting, formerly chief inspector of the Social Services Inspectorate, was asked to inquire and report on the management and practice of residential care nationally. Perhaps the most important outcome was that the Pindown report succeeded in focusing national attention and debate on the neglected issue of residential care.

___

The Pindown investigation was perhaps the best known, but it was just one of several mediums through which Barbara Kahan communicated her views during the 1980s and 1990s. From 1985 to 1994 she was chair of the National Children's Bureau and oversaw a wide-ranging review of its work. Her OBE in 1989 was awarded for services to the Bureau. As soon as the Pindown inquiry was completed, she was asked by the National Institute for Social Work to chair a multi-disciplinary group on residential care to take further issues that had been raised by the Wagner Development Children's Group (which she had also chaired). Drawing on the group's thinking, Barbara produced *Growing up in groups* which established a common core of residential practice applicable to children's homes, boarding schools, therapeutic communities and hospitals, and was sent to every SSD and social work training course and reprinted three times (Kahan, 1994).

Barbara did not remain aloof from children for in 1996 she became chair of a children's special needs boarding school. She endeavoured endlessly to raise the status of residential workers, to improve practice, to expand training and to demonstrate that residential care still had an important role to play in the care of children. Reluctantly, after many years of supporting joint training for field social workers and residential staff, she concluded that current training had failed residential workers. She advised that their training would have to be separate from social workers if their skills, specialist tasks and knowledge base were ever to be given the resources and attention they deserved.

By no means did Barbara limit herself to residential care. She identified a decline in child care practice as a whole within SSDs, much of which she attributed to the way the departments were and had been managed since the 1970 Local Authority Social Services Act. She made no secret of her criticisms, and said:

> After 1970 our vision of child care went out of the window. Today I am deeply concerned at some of the things which happen. Children in care now seem to have numerous changes of placements and the separation of siblings from each other has been much too common.

> The organisation of SSDs going generic overnight was ill conceived. It might have been better to have had a federation of social workers with specialists and some generalists but not to give every social worker mental health, the elderly, delinquents, fostering, adoption, everything to deal with at once. What better method could have been found to

destroy something? After further local government reorganisation, directors of social services have been at a height so far removed from the coal face that they have not been able to know what was going on in their departments.

The large organisations seem to have been less able to replicate the relatively firm corporateness of senior staff and practitioners working together with common standards and purposes as Children's Departments experienced. Everything seems so fragmented and good child care cannot be done in a fragmented way.

What is so sad about the present situation is that many staff seem to have no real sense of conviction about what can be achieved with children and young people. They have a feeling of working hard yet in some of my consultancy work I have found foster children among unallocated cases – even when caseloads are as low as 15-20 per worker. The hands-on staff often do not receive the professional supervision and support they need in the extremely difficult work they have to do, whether in group care or in field work of various kinds. Social work seems to have become more a job than a vocation. And there is a lack of leadership. It is very discouraging to see what has happened.

I must add that I believe that the people who are attracted to social work and residential care have as much capacity for commitment and vocational motivation as they ever had but they are not always best supported by the systems and structures in which they have to carry out their work. In consequence they may lack the job satisfaction which would help them sustain the inevitable stress and anxiety involved. Social work is among those occupations in which stress has greatly increased. I can only hope that with a change of political climate we may recover some of the optimism which is needed in such a difficult task. (Kahan, 1999, interview with author)

Barbara Kahan's achievements

Barbara spent a long time in the world of child welfare. When asked, 'What have you achieved?' she answered promptly and briefly:

First, I helped to personalise the Children's Departments. Second, I recruited some excellent people to the Oxfordshire Children's Department, some of whom went on to do much in social work. Third, I contributed to making policy makers more aware of the users of services. *Growing up in care* was a turning point. Fourth [and said with a gleam in her eye], the demolition of approved schools. (Kahan, 1999, interview with author)

Beyond doubt, Barbara was an outstanding if not *the most* outstanding children's officer. When she started the role as a young woman in Dudley, Children's Departments were not only new, they were even unwanted in some local authorities. The Devon Children's Department was larger than most yet, when Kenneth Brill started as its first children's officer, he was not considered worthy of a parking space. The explanation for this aversion was that some councillors and officials had wanted child care duties to be placed within existing Education or Health Departments. Within 20 years, Children's Departments had become the leading social work agencies, had influenced legislation and were the backbone of the new SSDs. Barbara was at the forefront of these advances simply because at Dudley and then at Oxfordshire she built up excellent departments with high standards of child care.

What was it that made her such a fine children's officer? Jean Packman said of Barbara:

She knew the job and had an enthusiasm which was conveyed to others so that the department became an exciting place to be. She worked extremely hard, came in early, was often the last person to leave. She was very strong in her beliefs and opinions. This caused arguments with people who disagreed but was stimulating for others. One result was that she attracted lively well-qualified people into the service. They were not toadies and had their own individual styles which Barbara allowed as long as children came first and if they worked all hours as necessary.

She was a hard taskmaster and could be very tough. When a teenage girl revealed that a head of a home had sexually interfered with her, he was gone immediately. There was no fudging, no doubting the girl's word, he was out. Anyone who exploited or damaged a child was a villain as far as Barbara was concerned. Her drive and convictions could come over as arrogance but it stemmed from a desire not for personal glory but from her determination to create a personal service that was the best for children. And it was personal. She frequently visited the children's homes. She insisted that Oxfordshire's children had the best, especially that they had a good Christmas. She would not let bureaucracy get in the way of children's relationships with her or with the child care officers. Simultaneously, she was always approachable and included her staff and students in her social life. (Packman, 1999, interview with author)

As an outstanding practitioner, Barbara Kahan could talk with authority. Subsequently, as a senior civil servant she succeeded in inspiring and stimulating myriads of welfare, educational and medical professionals. Not least, she then served as a pivotal figure in official committees and inquiries. All these provided her with the ammunition and status to be Britain's leading child care campaigner. On conference platforms, on television and radio, in numerous publications, she conducted a crusade for agencies which better served vulnerable children and their families. More than any other single person, she contributed to the reform of approved schools and their transformation as part of the 1969 Children and Young Persons Act. She was a leading voice and lobbyist in the movement which led to the formation of SSDs in 1970. The actual shape of the new organisations was not exactly as she had wanted, however, and later she was honest enough to acknowledge that some of the developments within the SSDs had actually harmed child care. In 1970, Barbara wrote that, as a result of the work of Children's Departments, "children now have greater importance in English national life than formerly" (Kahan, 1970, p 59). Over 30 years later, it is not too much to say that their importance has continued to grow and that much of the credit was due to Barbara Kahan.

Professor Roy Parker, a notable child care researcher, knew Barbara Kahan for over 40 years, and stated:

> Her contribution is immense. Once she starts she keeps with it until the bitter end. She is relentless and passionate. She is politically skilled, although she can be heavy-handed. I appreciate her because she was the first children's officer who said to me, 'I think research is valuable. I think what you are doing is valuable'. (Parker, 1999, interview with author)

Parker highlighted her virtue of persistence. In a similar vein, Terry Philpot, the long-serving editor and now editor-in-chief of *Community Care*, the leading social work magazine, pinpointed her painstaking attention to detail.

Recalling her contribution as a member of the Association of Children's Officers, he wrote that she was:

> ... willing to give 12 years service to her professional association, to put up with the long hard slog of committee work, to act as an adviser, to get down to the minutiae. What one sees in her writing is not so much the lofty phrase and noble sentiments of the reformer; they are there but in a secondary position, vastly overshadowed by a painstaking dealing of hard fact, turning over statistic after statistic and the careful dissection of themes and ideas. (Philpot, 1977)

It is the unusual combination of persistence, preciseness, political adeptness, practice and painstaking effort that has characterised Barbara Kahan. As Terry Philpot concluded,

> She is the Great Propagandist, the standard bearer *par excellence* in the children's cause – crusade might be a more apt description when one recognises the fervour with which the campaign has been waged ... none has beaten the drum of child care within the service more loudly. (Philpot, 1977)

Barbara Kahan died on 6 August 2000. Before she died, she read, corrected and approved this chapter. Her professional life span coincided with many major developments for disadvantaged and deprived children. She started work while Eleanor Rathbone was still battling for family allowances in the House of Commons. She knew Marjory Allen and was one of the main pioneers who put Lady Allen's vision of a personal service for children into action. Barbara Kahan stands with Eleanor Rathbone and Marjory Allen as a children's champion. But she was also a link between them and future progress. Marjory had foreseen the possibility of preventative work to stop children needlessly coming into public care but it was Barbara who introduced it to Oxfordshire and who campaigned to make it a national policy. Moreover, it was Barbara who took up Eleanor's early identification of the way in which poverty undermined family life. She therefore urged the reduction of poverty as an important part of any strategy of prevention. Barbara also went beyond Marjory in her detailed analysis of the dangers of and abuses within residential care while simultaneously making the case that residential establishments could be of help to some children if given proper resources and trained staff. Barbara, probably more than any other person, therefore ensured that residential care did not sink without trace by the start of the new millennium. Not least, Barbara had much closer contact with vulnerable children. She took homeless children into her home and, when she was a children's officer, sometimes had babies sleeping in her chest of drawers, because she could find no other placement for them for a night. She possessed a great gift of communication with children (and former children) in public care. She encouraged and enabled them to express their views. She thus played a part in a theme which grew progressively stronger from the 1980s: that users of services should help shape the programmes and policies which are supposed to help them. This interaction with children who were separated from their own parents probably also convinced Barbara of the vital importance to all children of their background or roots. This was a theme also highlighted by John Stroud, who is discussed in the next chapter.

FOUR

John Stroud, 1923-89

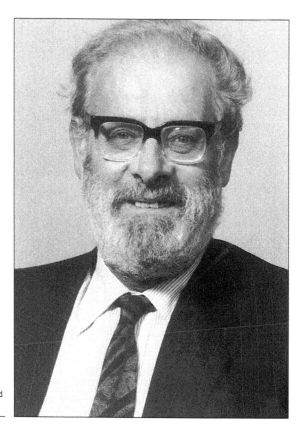

Photograph of John
Stroud, kindly supplied
by Daphne Stroud

In 1962, I started as a child care officer with Hertfordshire Children's
Department. I was informed that I would take over cases from John
Stroud, the boys' welfare officer who had been promoted. "You know
who he is, don't you?", said my senior officer. To my shame I did not.
"He's the novelist, he wrote *The shorn lamb*", she informed me, in reverential
tones. A few days later, John Stroud came to see me. He came into my
office and sat on the table, as the room was so small that it could take only

one chair. This was difficult for he was a large built man. Sensing my nervousness, he spoke kindly and talked about some of the boys I would be supervising. He then took me to visit a couple of children's homes. As we drove, his manner was mild, witty, almost zany, yet there was a certain hardness about him. At this time, he was already both a successful child care practitioner and a widely-read child care novelist.

Early life

John Stroud was born on 31 March 1923 in Maidstone, Kent. The lights in his street were still fired by gas and tradespeoples' horse-drawn carts were common. His father was a local government clerk, his mother a teacher who had been an active suffragette. John, a sister nine years older and a brother four years younger, had a comfortable upbringing. Indeed, when John was about six his mother had a small legacy and bought the family's first car: a Wolseley Hornet.

Mr and Mrs Stroud were keen amateur theatre and concert participants and performed with the Maidstone Dramatic Society. His father became well known locally as a producer and John frequently accompanied him to rehearsals and shows. In a private memoir, he recorded, "I liked theatre work and would like to have done more but I was much too shy, nervous and introverted to be any good on stage". He continued, "I was a solitary person. I did a great deal of reading and I invented and played many games on my own, and I daydreamed a lot. Much of my dreaming was about being in the theatre in one capacity or another. My other wish was to be a writer" (Stroud, undated, p 6).

As a child John spent little time roaming around with other children. Once his family bought a wireless set, he became a devotee of dance music, Children's Hour and the Saturday night serial, especially if it was by Charles Dickens. His mother frequently took him to the cinema where a film called *The gap* made a strong impression on him. The film was really a preparation for war: recalling the use of poison gas in the First World War and warning that, in the next war, the enemy would probably drop gas on Britain's civilian population. The film was forewarning that parents should be prepared for their children to be evacuated.

John started school when he was four, attending for two hours a day in a tiny class run by a Miss Emm in the front room of her house. He recalled, "I was at that time a withdrawn rather disturbed little boy. Already troubled by poor eyesight when very little and still in nappies.... I was very prone to having 'accidents' of various incontinent kinds. I had nightmares and more than once I walked in my sleep" (Stroud, undated, p 3). Eventually he won a place at the town's grammar school where his greatest pleasure was cricket. He played in the school first team for five seasons. In a match against the schoolmasters, he bowled a beauty which dealt the English teacher a painful blow in the crotch. The recipient was to achieve even greater literary fame than John: he was William Golding. By the time John was a sixth former, the Second World War had started and the cricket players sometimes stopped to watch aerial fights. On one occasion, waves of German bombers were being shelled by anti-aircraft guns. Four of the players, including John, refused to take cover. A large, sharp nose-cone of a shell fell within inches of them. Any closer and death would have been a certainty.

The Royal Air Force

In 1941, John Stroud left school and started work as a junior clerk in the county Education Department. Within a few months he was called up into the Royal Air Force (RAF) where his desire to be aircrew was ruled out by his poor eyesight. After the infantry training he was sent to Leighton Buzzard to be trained as a Clerk Special Duties (SDs). To his surprise, the small camp was completely camouflaged, and inside was an operations room. Radar was just being developed and Clerk SDs traced the course of enemy planes. Within a few months, John Stroud, just 18 years old, received orders for embarkation abroad. After a hasty goodbye to his girlfriend, he joined a huge convoy of ships heading for India. Near the end of the long sea voyage, he was taken seriously ill and was carried into Bombay on a stretcher. His temperature was so high that, later, nurses informed him that he had been near death. His illness was diagnosed as septicaemia and he took weeks to recover. These were unhappy weeks in which he felt weak and isolated.

At last he was deemed fit enough to re-join his draft at a camp near Madras, where he plotted whatever flights the somewhat primitive radar and radio systems could pick up. The most exciting event was seen to be the arrival of women, in the form of Eurasians of the Women's Auxiliary Corps India. A number of his colleagues became involved with the girls. John was much more involved in the camp concerts for which he wrote sketches and monologues. He eventually found the courage to go on stage himself, saying, "I could find a sort of protection in grotesque costumes. Once I was the hind legs of a pantomime horse and once a WAC(1) private and once an opera singer, but my part was principally to write the scripts" (Stroud, undated, p 15). He then wrote a small serious play which was broadcast over the local All-India radio. Soon he was writing radio scripts regularly, including a series about a detective called Hector Slaughter with airmen playing the main characters and John himself playing the minor ones. By 1944, he was ready to write, direct and produce his own pantomimes, one of which was attended by the Governor of Madras and his retinue. These successes benefited John in two ways. First, his self-confidence as a writer was boosted. Second, he found himself with a circle of friends. He celebrated his 21st birthday with a large, drunken party for friends who presented him with an engraved silver-plated cigarette case.

As more women were drafted into the camp at Madras, so the men were posted to the Burmese border where the Allies were fighting the Japanese. John's turn came in 1945 when he was transferred to Chittagong where he again organised camp concerts. But it was not all play, for the operations room was plotting all the air activity on the Indo-Burmese border. Next, John was posted to an island called Akyab from which the Japanese had just been driven. It was now used by American planes to drop supplies to troops operating behind Japanese lines in Burma and it was here that John first experienced bombing from Japanese planes. It was fortunate that few direct hits were received, for there was little shelter and the troops were living in tents. Not surprisingly, opportunities for concerts were few but John and a friend produced a magazine called *Present Tents.* With no access to printing facilities and only limited use of a typewriter, only one copy of each edition was produced. It was then passed from hand to hand until it disappeared. As the war drew to a close the British government began sending stars, such as Vera Lynn, to this hitherto neglected area. Under the grandiose title of editor of a magazine, John was even able to interview George Formby.

The time came for John to return to Britain. He was eager to return, but he realised that his years in India and Burma had had a profound effect on him. He had gained respect for Indian and Burmese people and was affronted by the racial prejudice of some armed forces personnel. He came across a paragraph in a newspaper about missionaries doing simple reconstruction work in Burma and wanted to do the same. He recorded, "I felt I wanted to leave the world a little bit better than it had been when I came into it" (Stroud, undated, p 21).

Back in Britain, John was posted to a RAF station in Essex. It was by now the glorious summer of 1946. He enjoyed the Essex pubs, travelled to London to see a test match at Lords, went to speedway at West Ham and to several theatres. He also took the opportunity to visit the good friends he had made during his service abroad. He travelled to Liverpool to be the best man at the wedding of one of his RAF chums in India, Phil Cain. Years later, Phil wrote:

> Freda and I went to meet him at Lime Street Station, Liverpool. I was on the lookout for him when I saw this gangling youth coming up the platform wearing a long white mac and a bush hat. He walked right up to us, never said hello, didn't give me chance to introduce Freda, and with that pulled an ocarina out of his pocket, and started playing it. You must remember that it was 1946, and people were giving us funny looks. (Tait, 1990, letter to Daphne Stroud, 28 January)

John sometimes said that he was a Goon before the Goons.

Unknown to John Stroud, this was also the period in which the Curtis and Clyde Reports were appearing, the reports which were to pave the way for the Children's Departments with which he was to be so closely associated. But, at this time, he was still serious about returning to Burma and decided that he would need some kind of qualification. At the camp, a resettlement officer told him about a two-year diploma at the University of Birmingham. After an interview, John was offered a place and in the autumn he donned his demob clothes of a sports jacket and flannels and made for the Midlands.

Into child care

In Birmingham, John lived as a student in an out-post of the Birmingham Settlement at Kingstanding. Its warden was Nancy Fear, who was assisted by two youth club leaders, a cook and five students. The other four students were girls; one was a shy student from Shrewsbury, Ruth Edwards. John and Ruth soon became engaged. He later wrote, "It wasn't a particularly sensible thing to do and I think that like many other youngish men at that time I was conscious of years lost to the War, and I wanted to catch up on life and not waste any more time. At any rate, I became engaged without ever being swept off my feet" (Stroud, undated, p 24).

During his second year, John went to the Colonial Office in London where an interview with "a large and formidable lady ... convinced me that the Colonial Service was not for me. I was simply not a smooth commissioned officer, public school type who could have become a District Officer barking out orders to the natives" (Stroud, undated, p 25). His decision not to return abroad was a relief to Ruth's mother who was not happy about the prospect of her daughter feeding a family on bowls of rice in the East.

Ruth's mother, who appeared to have a strong influence on John, also persuaded him to give up the diploma and to do a degree. John was reluctant to do the extra year which this entailed but admitted that, in terms of a career, a degree would be more useful than a diploma. The drawback was that he was not happy at university. He found he did not fit in well with other students who "were the children of well-to-do Midlands business people, and many of them had held commissioned ranks in the forces" (Stroud, undated, p 24). Further, he struggled with the academic subjects of a degree in commerce, particularly economics, which he failed twice. In 1949, when he was due to take his finals, he spent a lot of time in Maidstone playing cricket with his brother who worked for and was in the team of the local authority Roads Department. In June he married Ruth and soon afterwards was informed that he had gained a second class honours degree. The question then was what he should do in terms of a job. By this time John Stroud had read the Curtis Report and the 1948 Children Act had become law. He applied for and obtained the post of children's welfare officer with Middlesex County Council; he was 26. So John joined the Children's Departments which Marjory Allen had helped to create and in which Barbara Kahan was already a children's officer in charge of a large department.

John was placed in an office in Willesden and therefore qualified for the London weighting extra of £25 which brought his salary up to £475. On a low salary and with London experiencing a post-war shortage of housing, the Strouds found it difficult to find accommodation and ended up with one room and a kitchen in West Hampstead. When their son, Nick, was born, they were asked to leave and found a flat in Dulwich. Ruth was soon pregnant again and was unhappy in a cramped flat which they shared with a large rat – hardly the best companion for a small baby. The landlord asked them to leave and they had to move in with John's parents in Maidstone and John had to commute to London.

At least John enjoyed his job. He had expected to spend most of his time finding foster homes for children stuck in institutions. Instead his caseload was made up mainly of teenage boys who had grown up in care and were living in hostels or lodgings. One young man, Dennis, was to prove significant to John, as he recounts in his memoirs:

When I went to see him for the first time I found him sitting on the edge of his bed in a corner of a huge dormitory on the first floor. We had a desultory conversation for a few minutes – about his job and his finances, his friends and his hobbies: and then suddenly he interrupted me and burst out, 'Please can you tell me, sir – why am I here?' I was astounded and didn't know how to answer. He rapidly explained that he had no idea where he came from or whether he had any living relatives and he did not know for what reason he had drifted into a large hostel in South London.

In the end I said lamely that I didn't know – but that I would find out. I went back to the office and found his case file. It was an untidy, dog-eared file handed down from the old Public Assistance Department. I learned that when Dennis was born, his mother was a single girl who was a long-term patient in a mental hospital.

As soon as I could I went back to see Dennis. I felt very uneasy about telling him of such a grotty background and I wondered what terrible fears and anxieties I might be setting up in his mind. I had no text books to guide me and in the end I decided that honesty was the best policy, and that I'd better tell him the whole truth. And so I did. I put it over as kindly as I could, but all the same I expect it was rather bald and unvarnished. At the end of my account Dennis gave a big sigh and shook his head and said, 'Oh, thank you sir, that's much better than I expected'.

In this brief interchange, Dennis had taught me several important lessons. The first was simply the enormous importance to people separated from their families of information about their lineage and background. The second was that if such people are not given true information then they will invent stories to satisfy themselves, and their inclination will be to invent stories that are much more worse than the truth: often they will blame themselves and their own misdeeds for what has happened to them. They cannot really accept the enormity of being forsaken by their own parents.

It all comes down to questions that people in care and adopted people constantly ask themselves: 'Who am I? Why am I here? To whom do I belong?' (Stroud, undated, p 26)

Much as he liked his job, John had to look to move to an area where there was more chance of getting accommodation. Living with his parents was causing friction. Late in 1951, he applied for the post of boys' welfare officer with Hertfordshire Children's Department. He was interviewed by the children's officer, Sylvia Watson, whom he liked straightaway, and the chair of the children's committee, Lady Rosamund Gibbs. He was offered the job and told he would have to learn to drive – he passed his driving test at the first attempt. So John Stroud joined the county where he was to stay for the rest of his professional life.

Hertfordshire Children's Department

The Strouds were able to purchase a small cottage in the Hertfordshire village of Cottered. For John it meant a pleasant rural retreat where he played cricket for the village team, helped to organise the Coronation celebrations of 1953 and found time to be clerk to the Parish Council. Things were different for Ruth who by now had given birth to a second child, Ian, and found herself 'stuck' in a village with few facilities, no bus service and with an elderly neighbour who upset her with her malevolent grumbling. She was depressed and, it must be said, at times John was not sensitive to her needs. On the contrary, he complained about "Ruth's standards of housekeeping" (Stroud, undated, p 29). He does not record, however, what part he played in keeping the cottage clean.

Cottered was 14 miles from John's office in Hertford. He could not afford a car and his problem of getting to work was only solved when his mother bought him a motorised bicycle. He was responsible, alongside one other worker, for nearly all boys aged 11 and upwards in the large county. Visiting them all only became possible when the Children's Department provided him with a BSA motor bike. With the young people, John was drawn more intensely into helping them discover who they were. He went further and attempted to put them in touch with long-lost relatives. Children taken in the care of the Public Assistance Department had often been separated from their siblings and sent to other parts of the county with no effort made to maintain communication between them. John delved into the records and often arranged meetings between brothers and sisters and, in some cases, reunited them with parents. He recalled in his memoirs:

> One day I found a boy living in a hostel in Cambridge whose mother was still alive and living in Watford. I went to see the mother and asked

if she would like to have David home, and she said, 'Oh, is he all right? Oh, yes please, no one has ever asked me before'. I found many cases where children were desperate to seek out their parents of whom they had no recollections. (Stroud, undated, p 29)

John's colleague in working with the older boys was Allan Hanson, a cheerful character of whom John wrote, "in him I found another foil as I always seemed to need" (Stroud, undated, p 28). They put on sketches and monologues at the staff annual conferences. Together they went to meetings of the Association of Child Care Officers, otherwise known as ACCO. ACCO was started in 1949 and soon had recruited members. It proved to be an important body in that it gave members mutual support, spread good standards of practice, campaigned to improve conditions of work and lobbied government about child care policies. John Stroud had no great liking for meetings and conferences but he soon perceived that ACCO could be of importance to child care and so he supported it. John offered to produce its own journal under the title of *ACCORD*. The first copy came out in 1954 in duplicated form. However, the president of ACCO, Adele Toye, made John re-write the editorial as she considered it to be in poor taste. It proved popular and a year later came out in printed form thanks to the nearby Dr Barnardo's Printing School. Initially John did most of the writing; indeed some editions were entirely written by him using such pseudonyms as Barbara Cartwheel and Luke Smee. Gradually the heavyweights of child care began to pen their contributions including Barbara Kahan, Clare Winnicott, Donald Winnicott and Roy Parker. John edited it for 10 years, in which time it progressed from being a news sheet to a respected and widely read professional journal. As editor, John was also a member of the Association's publications and public relations sub-committee which, as well as over-seeing ACCO's publications, made contacts with many MPs in order to convey the views of child care officers. John was not at his best in networking with MPs and cabinet ministers, although at a later time he stood unsuccessfully as a Liberal parliamentary candidate.

In 1955, the Strouds moved to Welwyn Garden City. Here, John and Ruth and their growing family – they now had four children in all, Nick, Ian, Rosalind and Sylvia – had perhaps their happiest times. Welwyn Garden City was a pleasant environment with shops and schools near at hand. Their eldest son, Nick, in an interview with me, said about his early childhood with his father:

He was larger than life, an admirable father. We all respected him. He only had to look at you and you did what you were supposed to do. I found him friendly and helpful and he spent all the time with you that you wanted. He filled our lives with nice things to do. We went for walks and he would help us make things. He helped us make a morse code receiver and even if I knew only three or four letters, he could make up a long message with it. We never had trouble about knowing what to do. He was very affectionate with us. But as he got older, he got more immersed in his writing and did not show it so readily – but it was still there. I think my brother and I had the best of him because he was younger then and not so busy. We never saw much of his work colleagues but he was very proud of 'his' boys who were in care. Some of them had guitars and had formed a band and he took us to hear them. He was pleased to show us a bit of what he did in his job. Sometimes he brought back things they made for him – a lampstand, a box for jigsaw puzzles – and he brought them in with pride. (Stroud, N., 1999, interview with author)

In 1957, Brian Roycroft joined the Hertfordshire Children's Department in his first post. He was later to be a distinguished children's officer and director of a social services department. He got to know John very well both as a colleague and friend so his comments, made in an interview with me, are worth recording in some detail. By this time, John had been promoted and was to supervise Brian, who said as follows:

I remember our first meeting when I was appointed. This bear of a man said, 'You've taken on a tough job in this new town of Hemel Hempstead'. I just got a great feeling of warmth and protection from him. And that continued. He was personally concerned about me. The supervision usually took place in a pub where we stayed for ages, often until closing time. He would go over my records in immense detail, correct my grammar in his big, bold handwriting and making comments. He would challenge me by throwing out a question like, 'What's the longest period of time you spent with this boy?' It turned out to be when I had transported him from one place to another. 'Right, what did you do in that time? Did you waste time by just driving?' We had a series of conversations about case work in cars. He said that kids relaxed in cars, the sound of the engine, the countryside, they were the best times to get under the skin of the child. When I visited a boy in a children's home, he said I should not just speak with him in the sitting room, rather I was to take him to a cafe. He was a brilliant supervisor. The three lessons he taught me were these. One, to be totally focused on your client. Two, to create the right environment – it could be in the car, sitting on a swing in the garden. Three, not to ask leading questions but to let the child come at his pace. 'Don't crowd him' was one of his favourite sayings.

He was also kind to me outside of work and I went several times for meals with John and Ruth in Welwyn Garden City. They were pleasant times but a bit stilted. Having been in the RAF, I got the family an invitation to a flying display in Cambridgeshire. Ruth didn't come which surprised me. John seemed very close to the kids.

I also mixed with John at ACCO meetings. There were people in ACCO who couldn't get on with him because of his moods. He did not suffer fools gladly and he did not suffer those who were lazy. I don't remember him attending any of the big conferences at Swanwick. The best thing he did for ACCO was his writing, especially *ACCORD*. When we were lobbying for prevention, he came to the meetings at Barnet where we discussed what needed to be done. John then went away and wrote it and no editing needed to be done. (Roycroft, 1999, interview with author)

The writer

Writing was to be the turning point for John Stroud. A new secretary, Lorah Chesney, came to work for John and soon she was typing out *ACCORD*. John recorded, in what, unfortunately, were the last words of his personal memoirs, "Observing that I had a bit of writing talent she began putting gentle pressure on me. 'Why don't you write a proper book?' she asked, 'something to make me laugh'" (Stroud, undated, p 29). Her suggestion was to have profound outcomes. Probably John had been thinking of a book and his son Nick talks about a manuscript which was never published. However, he now got down to a book based on his personal experiences. Brian Roycroft recalls that "John gently revealed to me that he'd got this potential book. I saw some of the early chapters and I would say to him, 'That's too much like old so and so'. At the time, he had an absolute crush on one of the girls in the department. She was gorgeous. She is the love interest in the book. He had all these weird names but they were all actual names" (Roycroft, 1999, interview). The novel that followed was *The shorn lamb* published by Longmans Green (Stroud, 1960).

It was dedicated to the memory of John's parents who, by this time, had died.

The shorn lamb was an instant success. One reviewer even referred to John as the new Charles Dickens in that he revealed a world of deprivation which was hidden from the public at large. It was a Book Society choice and soon came out as a Penguin paperback. Later it was serialised on the BBC Radio 4's Book at Bedtime and on Woman's Hour. It sold well in English-speaking countries abroad and was on the syllabus of schools as far away as Australia and New Zealand.

The shorn lamb was by no means the first post-war social work novel. Joyce Carey's *Charley is my darling* (Carey, 1950) and Catherine Coles' *Michael O'Leary* (Coles, 1961) are both about underprivileged and 'delinquent' children. Yet they had nothing like the impact of John Stroud's book. On the surface it is a straightforward account of a newly trained child care officer, Charles Maule, and the young people on his caseload. These included Egbert Crump, who went rapidly through eight different placements; Sidney Smee, passive, inarticulate and delinquent; Donald Magoon; and Lennie Lumb. What made it so successful? For a start, it came out at an appropriate time. The welfare state had been set up and, indeed, was being much debated. The occupation of social work, particularly in child care, was expanding with many new college courses being established. A well-written social work novel was immediately seen as an ideal first book for students.

But it was not just that the book came out at the right time. It was an extremely well-written and well-crafted novel. It starts with Charles Maule (clearly based on Stroud himself) in his last lecture at his red-brick university. The (fictional) reader in social administration recounts the provisions of the 1948 Children Act and tells of the need for highly skilled child care officers to deal with the 80,000 children in care. Charles, who has already secured a job in a Children's Department, muses on his psychological knowledge – "perhaps leaning a shade towards Adler rather than Freud" (Stroud, 1960, p 8) – and takes satisfaction that he does possess the skills. In the next paragraph, he is thrown into the area children's office, has an orange box for a chair and is briefed by Miss Dashforth who "looked as though she had spent the last two months on some maniac task, such as trying to get a swarm of flies into a tea chest" (Stroud, 1960, p 8). He is rapidly introduced to the boys he is to supervise and suddenly his intellectual studies do not seem so useful. But Stroud's writing skills are such that the reader wants to know more about the young people. Their lives and

Charles' interaction with them are then interwoven, plus the bonus of his growing romance with one of the women child care officers.

The book was also realistic. Despite the strange names given to characters – Mrs Scatterbread, Paddy O' Hooligan, Mavis Nazimova Craggs and so on – anyone in the world of child welfare would have identified with the events. There are the foster homes that broke down just when the child care officer thinks they are going well; the emergencies that always happen at weekends; the court hearings at which well-to-do magistrates struggle to understand the likes of Egbert Crump of 6, the Rat Yard, Blight Street, charged with the theft of a budgerigar, and at which Egbert struggles to understand the language and formality of the legal system. Despite the pathos, the young people come over as real with deep emotions and needs which are not being met. And the book does not shy away from the failings of staff. The hostel warden is arrested for sexually abusing boys in his care; this is not a new phenomenon.

And the book was funny. When Sidney Smee is sacked by United Gnomes, he takes his revenge by scattering a dozen assorted pixies "all over the town in various grotesque, not to say obscene positions" (Stroud, 1960, p 124). John Stroud funnily and savagely describes the pretentious middle-class couples who want to foster a child but consider it beneath them to be questioned about their own backgrounds. In like manner, he laughs at A.J. Smurthwaite, the permissive head of the private special school, the Cottage in the Sun, who thinks classrooms are an out-moded convention and who specialises in Zoroastrianism – "'Did you see my article in last month's *Totem* – the one on Teen Age Fire Dancers?'" (Stroud, 1960, p 153). But he is also able to poke fun at himself. He asks the probation officer if he agrees that a boy's offences occurred because he "returns compulsively over and over again to his problem of non-existent Mother, creating and then shattering some symbol of her femaleness?". To which the down-to-earth Mr Bland replied, "No, old boy, I just think he's lonely" (Stroud, 1960, p 125).

John Stroud put his finger on a topic which was not only a concern for him, but which was also getting through to the public at large: the need for children in care to know about and to have contact with their relatives. Egbert Crump's mother neglected him, shouted and swore at him. But she stood up for him in court because she was his mother. Donald Magoon had not seen his mother since birth yet he always longs to be with her. Despite the objections of the superintendent of the home where Donald had been for years, Charles Maule somehow tracks her down and, on leaving care, Donald goes back to his mother.

Finally, the book was moving. Charles Maule faces despair, even wants to give up the job when another teenager turns to serious crime. Yet this is out-matched by the no-hoper who gels with elderly foster parents, and by Egbert Crump, who, as a stable young man, keeps in touch with his former child care officer.

Other novels followed. None were so successful as *The shorn lamb*. Nonetheless, *On the loose* (1961a), *Touch and go* (1961b), *Labour of love* (1965) and *Up and down the city road* (1968), sold well as they told about the lives of what were then called 'problem families' and of the staff who coped with them.

The success of his novels increased John Stroud's bank balance and the family moved to a larger house in Letchworth. But his marriage, which had been under threat for so long, finally fell apart. Nick Stroud talks sadly and perceptively about the break-up:

> My mother, Ruth, was very sweet. She worked hard to run the home and it was a struggle with four children and then a large house in Letchworth. She wanted everything to be nice and was much more focused on us. He was able to do so much because she did everything behind the scenes. He was very attentive to her in the early years but then he got much more sucked into his writings and work and she was left to look after us. I think it all went wrong when his writings did not bring him commercial success. He wanted to be a professional writer. He had a children's adventure story turned down. When he did not become a full-time writer, he just drove himself even harder and that got in the way of his marriage. He neglected everything, including his own health. They split in 1969. My mother adored my father and was very hurt. I was older, just going to university but I think it had a profound effect on my brother and one of my sisters. (Stroud, N., 1999, interview with author)

John and Ruth divorced in 1971. Ruth, with the girls, moved to Edinburgh where she embarked on a successful career as a social worker with the social work department. John married Daphne Pinkney in 1971 and lived in the village of Hertford Heath. I interviewed Daphne there in 1998, some nine years after John had died. She was keen to point out that her relationship with John did not develop until his first marriage was beyond repair. She had joined Hertfordshire Children's Department in 1963 as a secretary in the adoptions section. By this time John was moving up the career ladder and he had been appointed deputy children's officer in 1964. Daphne recalled that staff were in some awe of him but, despite his sarcasm, most found him easy to work with. When Lorah Chesney left, Daphne took over her post.

Daphne sometimes observed John with Nick, Ian, Rosalind and Sylvia and it is interesting to record her comments on John as a father, "He was a good father, avuncular in nature. But he did not express affection easily and was not tactile in the least. His novels are a bit sloppy and romantic but he was not at all like that" (Stroud, D., 1998, interview with author). I asked what he was like as a husband. Daphne laughed and replied, "Terrible, moody, he would go days without speaking". Yet obviously she had loved and admired him. She continued, "He was a perfectionist. He would not be worn down by anyone. He had tenacity" (Stroud, D., 1998, interview).

As John's secretary, Daphne had been willing to type his novels, his other books and his articles. All of this was with the permission of Sylvia Watson, the children's officer, who saw that John had a writing talent that had to be expressed. Yet it was on condition that he did not neglect his duties within the department and both Sylvia Watson, whom I had interviewed for a previous child care book (Holman, 1998), and Daphne Stroud were agreed that no one could accuse John of not fully carrying out his social work, administrative, practical and supervisory duties. Given that he carried out his tasks so fully, it is amazing that his writing output was so enormous. He was glad to hand over the editorship of *ACCORD* in 1965 but continued as a regular writer for the *Health and Social Services Journal*. He wrote a series of child care articles and then ghost stories for the *People's Friend*. He wrote a careers guide about child care, two guides for parents, and also made frequent broadcasts. He undertook historical research for his history of the Church of England Children's Society published by Hodder and Stoughton under the title *13 penny stamps* (Stroud, 1971). He edited and wrote in a very successful academic book called *Services for children and their families: Aspects of child care for social workers* (Stroud, 1973). In all, he wrote 14 books while his numerous articles cannot be counted. How did he do it? Daphne explained, "When he came home, he started writing. I was a writing widow. He wrote by hand, in ink, and hardly ever crossed anything out. He just wrote" (Stroud, D., 1998, interview).

John was addicted to writing. It was by pen that he best expressed his emotions, as he was not a great public speaker. I was present when he came back to Birmingham University as an after-dinner speaker. A large audience was anticipating the wit revealed in his novels, and the child care insights he displayed in his articles. He was nervous, almost shy, spoke too slowly, and read out every word as he peered through his thick spectacles. Brian Roycroft stated, "I heard him speak at a conference about communicating with children. He read it all, he was stiff, it was disastrous. Later I heard him at a seminar where he was much more at ease. It was smaller" (Roycroft, 1999, interview). On his feet, John had little of the passion and inspiration which Barbara Kahan displayed at numerous conferences. At his desk, pen in hand, he was funny and emotive. Similarly, as Daphne revealed, he was better in a small radio studio with no visible audience than he was on television where he tended to let other speakers grab the limelight. It was as if he had to have something between him and the audience. Even on stage, he did not appear as himself but invariably donned an outlandish costume.

Probably it did not matter that John was not a great speaker. The fact was that he could write. The other champions in this book have also written some significant, even outstanding books. John Stroud was different in that his writings reached such a wide range of people. His books were praised by academics, by historians, by social workers, and by reviewers in the quality newspapers. Yet he was also enjoyed by those who read the *People's Friend* and by the thousands who just wanted a good read. He wrote easily, powerfully, graphically and simply. It has been mooted that John should have concentrated on either child care social work or writing. After all, he never became a children's officer and he never became a full-time novelist, although he did apply for at least one post as a children's officer. He was not upset at not being selected – he was not keen to be the head of a huge SSD. The reason, I think, is that he was never completely at ease with what he called "the officer class" and, as the head of a social work agency, he would have had to mix socially with the aristocrats and the former public schools people on the committees. As Nick Stroud noted, he had hoped to be a professional writer. Brian Roycroft added, "He took great pride in his writing. He had a great skill and, in some ways, I reckon he thought he was in the wrong career" (Roycroft, 1999, interview). Yet I am not sure that his books would have been so successful if he had withdrawn from child care. His writings, fact and fiction, were mostly rooted in the world of welfare. It was his social work that gave him something to write about.

"His own branch of social work"

From his earliest days with Middlesex, John had identified the importance of family members maintaining links with each other. As a child care officer, he dealt with numerous cases of children who had been taken into public care and permanently separated from their parents. The separation had sometimes been the result of a deliberate policy in pre-war days in which the children were 'rescued' from so-called, inadequate, neglectful, cruel or immoral parents who were considered not to deserve to have the care of their offspring. Instead, the children were given a 'fresh start', away from the 'evil' influence of their families. By the time of the Children's Departments, staff may not have held these views but they were often just too busy to spend time tracing the parents of children who had settled into children's homes, or did not want to upset stable arrangements in foster homes.

John was one of the first child care officers to perceive that many separated children were both hurt and puzzled by their lack of knowledge about their backgrounds and by the absence of links with their parents and siblings. He led by example, ensuring that the children on his own caseload maintained contact with or at least had full knowledge about their own families. As he reached senior rank, he counselled the staff he supervised to do likewise. I was one of them, as I shall recount later. In time, his practice became policy in the Hertfordshire Children's Department. Sylvia Watson stated:

> ... you may replace a home but you still have this great desire to know where you come from and who you are ... a lot of time was spent in tracing who children were, who their parents were. We reunited quite a number. Often that meant just getting them to meet each other. Often it was mothers meeting illegitimate children: they could not keep them but, with a bit of help, they could have them home for a visit. My deputy, John Stroud, was very keen and did much of the tracing. To know in many cases, that they really had been loved but it had been impossible for mothers to care was a great comfort to the young people. (cited in Holman, 1998, p 103)

Somewhat to his surprise, John discovered that not only had siblings been separated from each other but even twins. Daphne Stroud recalled well that his first case involved two illegitimate girls taken from a Finnish mother during the Second World War. One girl subsequently discovered she was a twin but could get no further. John helped her to go to the High Court to obtain access to her papers. He realised that his seniority, status and expert knowledge could be of use to other twins. Such twins had not necessarily been taken into public care and often they had been placed for adoption. The common factor was that they had been separated and usually not informed that they were twins. His success prompted more, who were seeking their twin, to be referred to him. He never charged a fee and enjoyed the detective work involved, although it was often time consuming with meticulous searches through archives and registers. In all, he succeeded in reuniting around 50 pairs of twins. A number of them subsequently took part in research concerning the effects of nurture and nature at the University of Minnesota, and John was flown to Minnesota to act as a consultant. He not only traced twins: not long before he died, he found a 96-year-old mother for a 73-year-old 'child'.

John's pioneering work with twins was recognised publicly in two directions. He was placed on an advisory committee which led to legislation that gave adopted children the right to see their birth certificates at the age of 18. Then, soon after he retired, a Desmond Wilcox BBC TV documentary highlighted his work in reuniting twins. John never received any 'establishment gongs' in recognition of his work. Not that this worried him, for he did not have a high opinion of the establishment. But he did have the satisfaction of knowing that twins had been reunited, that the practice of separating twins had been stopped, and that he had contributed to the breaking down of the rigid secrecy surrounding adoption. As one journalist wrote after interviewing him, he is "The man who founded his own branch of social work" (Jervis, 1987).

When Children's Departments were abolished in 1970, John was one of the many child care staff who were incorporated into the larger Hertfordshire SSD. He was saddened when Sylvia Watson was not appointed as its director (she became the director in Cambridgeshire). She had handled John well, coping with his moods and encouraging his talents. She was an authority figure whom he respected and with whom he had a warm relationship. It is no coincidence that the Stroud's second daughter was named Sylvia. John became an assistant director in the new department but he was never at ease with it. Daphne Stroud said, "He did not like SSDs. He thought they drew in second rate people who took huge salaries but who were not really interested in child care. He was bitter about senior managers who left departments with golden handshakes without having contributed much. He made enemies because he did not conceal his views. Also some were jealous of him because of his successes outside the department and because of the publicity it attracted" (Stroud, D., 1998). Margaret Jervis, in an interview with him just after he retired, recorded along similar lines, "The post-Seebohm world of social work has held few attractions for the many strands of Stroud, drawing in, he thinks, too many second rate careerists. Seeing Seventies 'quackspeak' supplanted by eighties 'managementspeak', the state of social work has hardly been advanced, he believes" (Jervis, 1987).

John Stroud retired in 1986, at the age of 63, after 34 years' service with Hertfordshire. He continued to trace lost twins, was active in the Hertfordshire Alcohol Problems Advisory Service (which he had helped to found) and he liked to clear overgrown country paths. He continued his practice of writing every week to his children. Nick married, had children and a job in computers at Edinburgh University. The other three children all completed higher education and also moved into responsible jobs. Then, in 1987, while on holiday in Spain, John suffered a stroke which kept him in hospital for eight months and then confined him to a wheelchair. Initially, he could not move or even feed himself. But John was ever the writer and his mind remained active. The hospital was busy and noisy so, in his head, he composed an amusing article about it being built over a railway station and then dictated it to his wife. He was flown back to a hospital in Hertfordshire and there followed some painful times for him, Daphne and his children. In an unpublished article, which Daphne gave to me, he wrote about, "my tendency to burst into tears for no apparent reason. A doctor told me that one part of my brain which had been damaged was that which controlled my emotional responses. I would burst into tears usually on happy occasions" (Stroud, 1988). He underwent much physiotherapy as he attempted to learn again how to control his speech and muscles. He recorded:

> My wife was a great help. She had taken the advisory booklets to heart, tried to do as little as possible for me, making me face the fact that it was I and I alone who had to do the work. She was particularly strict if I whined about my lot. Her attitude led me into mixed feelings – I felt ambivalent, appreciating intellectually what she was doing but irrationally resenting what she was saying.

> My family did, later, have cause to complain of my testiness and flashes of ill-temper. I found a sort of antidote in writing and from about the fourth month after the stroke I entered a period of surprising productiveness. No masterpieces emerged, but I did, at least, get on top of my muddled mind for a while. Sometimes the simple rhythms and rhymes of poetry imposed order. (Stroud, 1988)

John refused to be housebound. He continued to work for charities, particularly those for deprived and disabled children and deaf people. As he could no longer manage stairs, Daphne moved his bed into the downstairs office where he did so much of his writing. It was here that he died on 31 August 1989.

A complex character

All human beings are complex, yet John Stroud was especially so. The extremes of introversion and extroversion were very apparent in him. At social gatherings, where people wanted to converse with the famous author, John Stroud, his big frame, clothed in a crumpled suit, might be found shuffling around the edges as he stared into his tea cup. The same John Stroud would dress in tights and ballet dress and have an audience of child care officers in near hysterics with his performance as the Sugar Plum Fairy. He avoided attention yet lapped up the applause. Brian Roycroft pointed out that he was not clubable and not sociable. John sometimes organised cricket matches against local approved schools in which Brian, no mean player, would participate. He smiled as he said, "He was captain, of course. He took it very seriously. But there was no socialising afterwards. The team played then went home" (Roycroft, 1999, interview).

He had a fine intellect and Margaret Jervis wrote that "his clarity of vision and purpose is simply the mirrored surface of a depth of intellect and roundness of character all too rare in public service today" (Jervis, 1987). John knew – and at times made it clear that he knew – that his understanding of social work and his commitment to child care was above that of many of the young managers who came into social services in the 1970s and 1980s. Yet he was not prepared to apply to be a director of social services where his abilities would not only have been useful but in which he could have challenged some of the directions in which social work was going in the 1970s.

The extremes of kind compassion and cheerfulness and ugly rudeness and gloom co-existed in him. As a child care officer, he would spend hours of time and effort with and for some dishevelled, withdrawn, unhappy and ungrateful teenager. He stuck with them with that tenacity that made him stick, for example, at the task of finding a lost twin. He was often gracious and supportive to his colleagues. Yet there was also the depression, the sharp tongue and the effective 'put-downs'. Brian Roycroft remembered:

He used to get black moods and periods of despair. We would go to the pub and I wouldn't get a word out of him. I'd try to get a conversation going and he would suddenly say, 'Don't crowd me'. Years later I was in a discussion group and John was sitting there and not making one contribution. I tried to involve him and he snapped my head off in front of everybody. Afterwards, Sylvia Watson told me not to worry about it. She was brilliant with him. She played him like a violin. (Roycroft, 1999, interview with author)

At one committee meeting of ACCO, its new president made a bombastic and inappropriate speech. There followed a prolonged silence until John, who had been sitting on a tiny chair in a corner, stood up raised his arm, bellowed "Sieg Heil" and sat down. Perhaps this particular deflating of pomposity was justified. At other times, his dark moods and sarcastic words were directed at the innocent. Not surprisingly John brought out extreme reactions in those around him. Some openly disliked him and saw him as arrogant. Others admired and almost loved him and were loyal to him.

Outside of his personal relationships, John Stroud's heart was in child care. Here he must be remembered for three main reasons. First, he played his part in establishing child care as a profession. To him, 'profession' did not mean a small, self-preserving, highly qualified elite. John Stroud, like the majority of the children's champions, never possessed what was recognised as a professional qualification in child care. By 'profession' he seemed to mean people with a commitment to deprived children, skills for working with them, and shared beliefs about the value of and the rights of such children. ACCO, which he supported for so long, was a mechanism whereby child care officers encouraged each other, where they exchanged information about their departments and where they promoted national policies which served the interests of deprived children and their families. John backed ACCO as it lobbied for legislation to legitimise and expand preventative action which would stop children unnecessarily being removed from – and so having their links cut from – their natural families. *ACCORD* became a forum in which child care issues were debated, theories expounded and new practices examined. It must be noted again that child care had not always been regarded as a specialist occupation or profession. Prior to 1948, statutory child care duties had been carried out by departments whose main function was schooling, health, destitution or even pensions. Some members and officials of these departments had resented the formation of Children's Departments and wanted to take back their child care duties. John Stroud was one of those who resisted such a backward step and insisted that child care had to be a specialist occupation in its own right.

John never claimed to be an academic. Sometimes he would laugh about his student days as evidence that he was not an intellectual. Yet *ACCORD* soon found a place in every child care library. Further, *Services for children and their families* was on the reading list on every social work training course in colleges and universities in the early 1970s (Stroud, 1973). So John Stroud also contributed to the training of students. By the time this book was published, child care officers had become social workers within the new SSDs. He was keen that their identity and specialist child care skills would not be lost and he wrote in the book's introduction:

> This book is therefore an attempt to record the position achieved by the child care service on the eve of reorganisation. It has been written by people who have been active in the child care service and have gained their experiences and formed their opinions in the thick of the fray. (Stroud, 1973, p ix)

He was somewhat afraid that the occupation of child care would be watered down. Whether that has happened or not is another matter. What can be recorded is that John Stroud was a pioneer who helped to establish child care work as a bona fide part of social work alongside the more traditional wings of probation, medical social work and psychiatric social work.

Second, he was one of the first practitioners to write about the needs of children in care to possess knowledge of and to maintain contact with their relatives. In expanding this kind of work to reuniting twins, he did, indeed, found "his own branch of social work". Historically, John Stroud was important for making the claim and spreading the message that the interests of most deprived young people was best served by maintaining their links with their birth families. From the 1970s onwards, child care social work was to be divided between those who accepted Stroud's view and those who emphasised permanently cutting children's ties with their kin if it gave them greater stability.

But he was not just adept at identifying and writing about the needs of deprived young people. He was also skilled at the practice of relating to them, their foster parents and, if possible, their biological parents. As mentioned, at times John did have difficulties in communicating with officials and others whose positions owed more to their educational and social privileges than to their abilities. By contrast, he was at his best with those who were then called the clients of the Children's Departments. As a young child care officer, I accompanied John Stroud on visits to clients. He was relaxed, attentive, concerned, understanding and, above all, had the knack of getting others to talk – no easy task with some sullen teenagers. On reflection, I decided that his expertise sprang from his own experiences and struggles. In his younger days he had felt solitary and isolated. As an adult he went through dark moods and flashes of anger which he did not fully understand. He had suffered the breakdown of a marriage. He therefore had an empathy with clients since, in some ways, he had stood where they were coming from. The outcome was a commitment towards their well-being which made him work tirelessly on their behalf. Often when social workers climb up the management ladder, they move away from face to face practice with clients. It is a tribute to John Stroud that, even when a deputy children's officer and assistant director, he still worked to reunite relatives.

Third, John Stroud did more than any other person to popularise child care, that is, he took the little known Children's Departments to the public at large. During the 1940s and 1950s, there were people who still remembered the war-time evacuation officers who found homes for evacuees. No doubt many would have heard of Dr Barnardo's in the voluntary sector and probation officers in the statutory sector. Few would have heard of child care officers. After all, Children's Departments were not established until 1948 and they were among the smallest local authority departments. John's novels brought child care to a larger audience. His books were not restricted to the academic few nor the literary elites. He reached the kind of people who went to free public libraries to borrow a novel which immediately won their interest, which moved their emotions, and which made them smile. The readers got their heart-warming stories and in reading they also learnt something about why children were removed from their parents, how it affected them, and how child care officers and residential staff were trying to help them. Nick Stroud commented about his father's novels, "He wrote about kind, generous and hardworking people giving up their lives to do good to children. He was taking things out from under the carpet and putting them in public view and saying, 'It's not so bad'. Today social workers get so much bad publicity" (Stroud, N., 1999, interview). John's novels, along with his articles in popular magazines and his broadcasts, must have made many people more sympathetic towards the staff and clients of Children's Departments. When I went to a party or some other social occasion, I did not try to hide my occupation, I was not ashamed of being a child care officer. It is a different story today when social workers tend to be unpopular. My experience is that the residents of inner city areas and council estates often regard them – wrongly in my view – as the officials who swoop in to take children away. Hence they are not welcome. Yet if they fail to remove children who then suffer abuse or neglect at home, the same social workers are condemned by the press for being too soft and permissive. Again, when social workers appear in TV soaps or plays, they are often portrayed in an unsympathetic and inaccurate light. As Mary Hartley, who has tried in vain to launch a realistic soap about social work, wrote, the "root of the matter ... is embedded in the public dislike and disdain of social services and the appalling public image of social workers" (Hartley, 1999). So poor is the image of social work, that applications to training courses have fallen to an all-time low. It would not solve the problem but it would certainly help if social work had a John Stroud today.

To my knowledge, John's last written words were a poem written in 1989. He was saying goodbye and it is appropriate that, to the end, he had happy thoughts about children:

> This is farewell to the dear dear lands,
> For I am disabled and I am grown old.
> I can no longer walk through the fields of gold,
> Or go to the mountain tops or the shore,
> Seeing the houses and farms nevermore;
> There'll be no more long days under the sun.
>
> Explorations of quaint little towns: these are done.
> Maybe I can hope that one day for an hour
> I may walk with my children and smell wild thyme in flower.
> One throat-catching hour at noon would be best,
> Before the sun sinks for all time in the West.
>
> (Stroud, 1989)

FIVE

Clare Winnicott, 1906-84

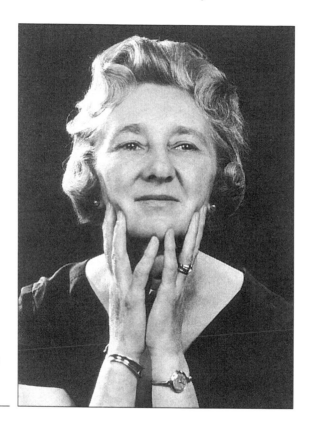

Photograph of Clare
Winnicott, kindly
supplied by George
and Janie Thomas

While Marjory Allen spearheaded the campaign which established local authority Children's Departments, Barbara Kahan was actually one of the children's officers who successfully organised them. John Stroud spread understanding of the 'new' child care to the public, and Clare Winnicott was the leading figure who trained staff for the child care service. Clare wrote just one book and very few articles. Even within these, she says little about herself. There is no published biography about her. Yet she was a charismatic person who made a strong impact on those who met her, and I was one of them. It has taken an American academic, Dr Joel Kanter, to gather material about Clare. He has not, as yet, published his book on Clare, yet he has most generously allowed me to see and to use his manuscript. Dr Kanter gives particular attention to Clare's interest in psychoanalysis and her editing of her husband's writings, whereas I will concentrate on her child care career. I wish to acknowledge that my account of Clare's early life relies very heavily on my conversations with Dr Kanter and on his draft manuscript (Kanter, undated).

A Baptist background

Elsie Clare Nimmo Britton (referred to hence as Clare) was born in Scarborough on 30 September 1906. Her father, James Nimmo Britton, a Glaswegian working man, had converted to the Baptist faith and he later became a minister. After two successful ministries in Lincolnshire, he and his wife, Elsie Clare, moved to Scarborough in 1903. By 1912, the family were living in Clapham, London, where the energetic Reverend Britton soon doubled the size of the congregation. Later they moved to Southend-on-Sea to Avenue Baptist Church, which was considered one of the leading Baptist churches in Britain.

James Britton's first sermon at his new church was based on Dr Livingstone's famous words, "Anywhere so long as it is forward". He put the saying into practice and became a well-known and popular minister in the town and beyond. He preached for conversions and the membership and the activities of the church multiplied. But his evangelism was not of the kind that made the congregation into a 'holy huddle', separated from other people. He encouraged the young people of the church to raise funds in order to bring underprivileged children from East London to Southend-on-Sea for a holiday. In addition, 1,500 low-income women from East London were transported in for a dinner and day's outing. During the General Strike in 1926, James Britton drew into the church both those who supported and those who opposed the strikers, and preached "What shall it profit a man if he gain the whole world and lose his own soul". When Southend began to feel the effects of the economic depression, he opened the church facilities to unemployed men and appealed to his congregation to find them jobs. He worked unstintingly, suffered two illnesses, and had to retire in 1935.

Clare's mother was the daughter of the Reverend William Slater, also a Baptist minister, who, in the Nottinghamshire area, had sided with the coal miners in their struggle for better conditions. She went to a teaching training centre in Nottingham; Dr Kanter believes it was the same one attended by D.H. Lawrence and two of his lovers. Certainly, she found Lawrence's sexual morals to be repugnant (Kanter, undated), and throughout her life she conveyed the notion of virtue to her children. Indeed, she may have communicated it so repeatedly that Clare later reacted against it.

Clare enjoyed an emotionally secure and happy childhood and, not surprisingly, was soon participating in church life where she was a Sunday School teacher and a leader of the Girls' Life Brigade. After attending High School in Southend, from 1929-30 Clare became a student at Selly Oak College, a Christian teachers' training centre in Birmingham. On leaving the college, she did not teach but spent much of the 1930s as a youth club leader with the Young Women's Christian Association in Nottingham and Norwich. By all accounts, she possessed a sparky and enthusiastic personality which, with her love of outdoor pursuits, would have made her an ideal club leader. Clare had clearly taken on much of her parents' concern for underprivileged families. This always remained with her but, at some point around this time, she parted company with Christianity and declared herself to be an atheist and socialist.

In 1937, Clare made her first contact with an institution which was to play a major part in her life: she went to the London School of Economics and Political Science (LSE) as a student on the one-year social science course. On completion, she obtained a post with the Commissioners for Special Areas as a club organiser for unemployed juveniles in Merthyr Tydfil. The Commissioners had been appointed for those areas particularly hard hit by the economic slump of the mid-1930s. Merthyr Tydfil was recognised as one of the most deprived areas in Britain and Clare also administered the Mayor's Boot Fund which provided footwear for unemployed miners and their families. Handing out boots to children made a lasting impression on her and, after the war, I remember her saying in a lecture that the welfare state had, at least, made that fund no longer necessary.

Clare Britton's involvement in youth club work, her concern for deprived areas and her allegiance to socialism reflected a person who wanted to improve the environment of poor people. It was at this stage that she also developed her interest in individual and family functioning. In 1940, by which time the Second World War was under way, Clare returned to the LSE to study social work on the 13-month mental health course. The course was considered to be Britain's leading training for psychiatric social workers and it is worth noting that her own study of individual and family dynamics started here, before she met some of Britain's leading psychiatrists later on in the war. When German bombing of London intensified, the course was suspended and then relocated to Cambridge. It was directed by Sybil Clement Brown, an eminent, imposing, yet kindly social work leader, who was later to be a member of the Curtis Committee. As well as attending lectures, the students undertook two practical placements. Clare's took her to the Oxford Child Guidance Clinic and then to the Mill Hill Emergency Hospital, London, where the students worked with adult psychiatric patients. During this placement, Clare became used to running to the air raid shelters when the sirens warned of imminent raids.

The course was small, with 12 students, most of whom were experienced social workers and capable students. Clare, now in her early thirties, was not outshone. Her academic brilliance was such that she not only passed, but also gained a distinction in, every subject. Her achievement was all the more notable in that she had not taken a degree at a prestigious university and she had not previously worked in a child guidance clinic, which was considered to be the top social work agency. Her success was due to her hard work, enthusiasm and ability.

The evacuation and Oxfordshire

Like a number of other children's champions featured in this book, Clare Britton's career and personal life was to be greatly influenced by the evacuation of children during the war. As a social worker with the magic PSW (Psychiatric Social Worker) next to her name, she could have taken a post in a sheltered child guidance clinic. Instead, she opted to be in the thick of the evacuation. Initially she worked with evacuation schemes in Reading and the Midlands. While at the latter, where she was employed by the regional health authority, she was sent to Oxfordshire, which had received many evacuees, to help on a part-time basis.

With thousands of children taken from their families and neighbourhoods, it was not surprising that some did not settle into their foster homes (or billets as they were sometimes called). In my book, *The evacuation: A very British revolution*, I explain how the government funded local authorities to set up over 200 hostels in England and Wales to take in such children (Holman, 1995, pp 122-4). These 'difficult' children were defined by the Ministry of Health as those "who, through difficulties of behaviour or temperament, could not suitably be billeted but needed a period of special care or supervision" (Ministry of Health, 1944, p 2). The Ministry added that the main problems of the children were stealing, enuresis and unruly behaviour. The hostels often had to rely on inexperienced and unqualified staff to cope with sometimes very demanding children. In Oxfordshire, the local authority appointed a child psychiatrist to work one day a week with the children and staff in its five hostels.

The psychiatrist was Donald Woods Winnicott; later he and Clare were to marry. Winnicott was born in 1896 in Plymouth to a wealthy and influential family. His father was a successful businessman and a Lord Mayor of Plymouth who was subsequently knighted. Like Clare, he had a religious upbringing, as his parents were devout Methodists; and like her, he later cut his links with the church. After public school, he studied medicine at Cambridge. In 1923, he became a physician at the Paddington Green Children's Hospital where, as a paediatrician, he became particularly concerned for patients in poverty. By the mid-1920s, he had taken up psychoanalysis. At this time he married Alice Taylor, of whom little is now known except that she was probably a professional musician. Michael Jacobs, who has written a biography of Winnicott, indicates that she "went mad" and that Donald had to care for her (Jacobs, 1998, p 12). By the late 1930s, Winnicott was an eminent figure in psychoanalytic circles and in December 1939 he joined with John Bowlby and Emanuel Miller to write a letter to the *British Medical Journal* in which they warned "that evacuation of small children without their mothers can lead to very serious and widespread psychological disorder. For instance, it can lead to a big increase in juvenile delinquency in the next decade" (Bowlby et al, 1939). They urged that the evacuation schemes should take into account the emotional needs of the children. Donald Winnicott made regular broadcasts with the BBC to give advice and reassurance to parents who had been parted from their children and to the foster parents who received them.

Donald was appointed psychiatric consultant to the government evacuation scheme in Oxfordshire. Once he started working, he perceived that the children taken in by the hostels were there not just because of the evacuation, but also because of unsatisfactory experiences within their own homes. He also observed that external factors, such as the atmosphere and the routine of the hostels, could have a profound impact on the children. This was to alter his therapy with children and, as Jacobs points out, distinguished him from his colleague Melanie Klein who concentrated almost exclusively on the "inner reality" of children (Jacobs, 1998, p 17). Winnicott enjoyed helping the children directly but soon decided that the most effective use of his time was to act as a consultant to the staff who had the everyday care of the youngsters. Until then he had not worked closely with social workers and, indeed, was regarded by some in

children and sometimes staff who felt they could not cope. She was called out at night concerning boys who ran away and once when a warden's wife ran away with the assistant warden. On one occasion, she was phoned by a warden asking what to do about a boy with suicidal tendencies who had climbed on to the roof. Clare swiftly advised that the boy be ignored. In short, Clare backed her own judgement in taking a risk and the boy came down. It had been up to Clare to make this decision among many others and, although Donald Winnicott wrote much about the hostels, she was the leading figure. Unfortunately, she received much less credit for the Oxfordshire scheme than Dr Winnicott.

The trainer

Soon after the end of the war, Clare spent some time looking after her seven-year-old niece and five-year-old nephew; they were the children of her brother, Karl, and his wife, who had been hospitalised for the birth of their third child. In her lectures, she sometimes referred to their antics to illustrate a point. She was also close to her brother, Jimmy, who had spent much of the war in German-occupied Crete, and her sister, Liz. Her siblings, too, were able people whose interests often coincided with hers. Karl became a professor of philosophy, Jimmy was a distinguished academic who studied language and wrote poetry, and Liz was an art teacher with an interest in how children expressed themselves through painting. Clare enjoyed the company and love of her family, and she also valued the love of Donald Winnicott. The latter was unhappily married; it is impossible, however, to be precise about when he and Clare became romantically involved.

Meanwhile, Clare continued to work in Oxfordshire where she retained responsibility for those evacuees who remained in the hostels after the war and where she also extended her child care range to cover foster care and adoption. At some point she also undertook resettlement work for the War Office for soldiers who had endured terrible times as prisoners-of-war. This experience, although short, clearly had a strong effect on her and years later she still talked about it in her lectures. By 1946, she had changed jobs and at a child guidance inter-clinic conference in November of that year the chairperson introduced her as having "recently joined the staff of the National Association for Mental Health and has become a member of the staff of the Education Department, dealing particularly with the findings of the Report of the Curtis Committee" (National Association for Mental Health, 1946, p 29).

During the post-war years, Clare Britton was a well-known social work figure. The work of the residential hostels had gained much attention, partly because the Ministry of Health had conducted and published a survey of their outcomes (Ministry of Health, 1944). The Oxfordshire hostels were particularly well known. According to Donald and Clare's writings, only a dozen of the 285 children in the Oxfordshire hostels had absconded and the vast majority had been settled into a stable environment; delinquency had been prevented; and "a fair proportion were brought to a much improved psychological condition" (Winnicott and Britton, 1947). Clare later pointed out that she had communicated the lessons of the hostels' work to committee members, local authority administrators, parents and the public. She added that, "It was the dissemination of this kind of first-hand knowledge from evacuation areas all over the country that eventually provided the momentum for the setting-up of a statutory committee of enquiry into the care of children separated from their parents [the Curtis Committee] and eventually led to that landmark in the social history of this country – the Children Act 1948" (Winnicott, 1984, p 4). She was called to give oral and written evidence to the Curtis Committee and she was in demand as a child care teacher at evening courses and conferences. She was, therefore, a significant figure on the child care scene when the late 1940s brought radical changes.

In her campaigns for reform of the child care services, Marjory Allen was critical of the lack of training among residential staff. When the Clyde and Curtis Reports appeared in 1946, they made the case for training, not just for residential workers but also for the field staff who the report referred to as 'boarding-out officers' (later called child care officers). The Clyde Report regretted that the boarding-out officers often lacked the skills to select and support foster parents and that residential establishments were dependent on nurses and people with no qualifications. It recommended "That there should be increased training in Child Care Work and further qualifications possessed by the Staff of Homes" (Scottish Home Department, 1946, recommendation 15).

The Curtis Committee dealt with the issue of training in even more detail. Indeed, it considered it so urgent that it issued an interim report urging the establishment of a Central Training Council in Child Care to promote new training courses for residential staff. In its full report, the Committee attributed many of the deficiencies of the child care system to a lack of trained staff and, in Appendix 1, recommended not just that boarding-out officers should be trained but also detailed the elements of their courses (Home Office et al, 1946, Appendix 1, para 1). It argued that courses for both field and residential staff should be organised by the Central Training Council in Child Care and should be "of university standing" (Home Office et al, 1946, Appendix 1, para 4). It acknowledged that field and residential staff should study some subjects in common but added that the former "would be taken on a considerably higher academic level" (Home Office, Ministry of Health and Ministry of Education, 1946, Appendix 1, para 4).

The government responded speedily. In 1947 (the year before the Children Act), it established the Central Training Council in Child Care and courses were started. Those courses for residential staff were located mainly in polytechnics and technical colleges while those for boarding-out officers were at the universities of Birmingham, Cardiff, Leeds, Liverpool, Nottingham and the LSE. Separate arrangements for courses were made in Scotland. When the legislation did go through Parliament, it did not specify that all the staff of the new Children's Departments had to be trained. Given that the services were expected to function almost immediately and given that so few existing staff possessed qualifications, such a requirement would have been impossible to achieve. However, the 1948 Children Act did specify that central government could finance courses and that grants would be available to students. The expectation was that Children's Departments would be run by an increasing number of qualified practitioners.

The tutors for these new courses were drawn mainly from graduates who had been active in evacuation schemes and from psychiatric social workers. In 1947, Clare Britton was appointed as tutor in charge of the child care course at the LSE. It was a one-year course and intended mainly for graduates. The students attended lectures – which included child development, sociology, the law and child care practice – and tutorials at the LSE, and went on practical placements in social work agencies. The tenor of their theory and practice was much influenced by the teachings of the two psychiatrists, John Bowlby and Donald Winnicott. John Bowlby's studies emphasised the crucial importance to children of a close, warm relationship with a mother or mother substitute. Donald Winnicott gave some lectures on the course, and his many articles and books gave much attention to the needs of deprived and disturbed children. Initially, the course was small in numbers, about 12 at the beginning, and the student group became close, supportive and Clare knew them all well.

These years were among the happiest in Clare's life. In 1951, Donald Winnicott and his first wife were divorced and by the end of the year he and Clare were married. She was 45 to his 55, and he had already suffered two heart attacks, although the difference in age and his health problems did not stop them enjoying a loving and fulfilling marriage. Clare was very happily married to Donald, but it has to be said that their relationship was one in which his reputation tended to overshadow much of her achievements. The LSE child care course was held in high regard, with its students eagerly sought by Children's Departments. Clare was in demand as a conference speaker and, in 1954, gave a paper at the United Nations Seminar on European Social Services. Yet the course disappeared as a separate entity in 1958. A number of social work leaders, particularly Eileen Younghusband, argued that the various branches of social work – such as child care, probation,medical social work, mental health and welfare – shared common values, theoretical foundations and objectives. This group, therefore, lobbied for common or generic training. The LSE obtained a grant to start a generic course in 1954, the applied social studies course for which Clare taught a child care component. She accepted that the various branches of social work did have much in common but she also maintained that each required very specialised knowledge and skills which could only be acquired on intensive, specialised courses. Donald backed her, drawing on his own clinical practice and many contacts with the child care services to make clear that professionals dealing with children required high levels of child care skills. Clare also found an ally in Kay McDougall. Like Clare, she had been brought up with strong values, was a socialist, had trained at the LSE, and was a psychiatric social worker. She headed-up the specialist mental health course at LSE and in 1954 founded *Case Conference*, the leading social work magazine. Kay was keen to advance a unified social work profession but believed it should retain a specialist element. As the grant for the generic course drew to an end, senior staff at the LSE had to decide how limited resources could be spent.

David Donnison, later one of Britain's most eminent and influential social policy professors, came to the LSE in 1956 as its new reader in social administration. The head of department, Richard Titmuss, asked him to spend time with the three courses and their leaders and to make a recommendation for their future. In an interview with me, David recalled:

> There were three courses, the child care course led by Clare Winnicott which had Home Office backing, the mental health course run by Kay McDougall with Ministry of Health backing and the generic course under Eileen Younghusband and funded by the Carnegie Trust. Clare was a creative, thoughtful woman who knew all the American

psychiatric stuff but never lost sight of the fact that she was training people for a public service. All three were remarkable women. I did recommend that there should be one amalgamated course because social work in Britain was coming together, would be integrated. I backed Kay as leader because she was a natural team leader but I warned that the other two might leave. (Donnison, 2000, interview with author)

Unfortunately, Clare was absent with meningitis during the crucial part of 1957 when decisions were made. Richard Titmuss consequently announced that the child care course would have to be integrated into the generic course (applied social studies). At a stroke, Clare lost her position of leading the foremost child care course in Britain. She was deeply hurt and upset.

Clare continued, however, to teach the child care theory and practice within the applied social studies course. Brian Roycroft met her during this period, when he was an assistant area children's officer with London County Council. He said in an interview with me:

I got the task of organising the student placements from the LSE and Clare involved me in the course. I did not find her easy to get on with at first because I was in awe of her. She was a formidable figure. But she was very kind. I was due to speak at one of the meetings and she realised that I was very nervous, not having done it before. She took me for a meal beforehand, went through my notes with me and was very encouraging. (Roycroft, 1999, interview with author)

With a reduced administrative load, Clare was able to give more time to training she had started at the Institute of Psycho-Analysis which included being analysed by the famous child psychiatrist, Melanie Klein. According to the study by Dr Kanter, their relationship was never an easy one, with Clare complaining about Klein's negative approach and lack of personal civility (Kanter, undated, p 42). Nonetheless, Klein did recommend that she should qualify as a psychoanalyst in 1960. Married to Donald, who served his term as president of the British Psycho-Analytical Society, Clare mixed frequently with Britain's top psychiatric figures. Yet, as Kanter makes clear, it did not dominate her social work life and some of her close colleagues at the LSE were unaware that she was undergoing analysis (Kanter, undated, p 38). Certainly, in her lectures, although she made reference to psychoanalytic doctrines, they were not the core substance of what she taught.

By the mid-1960s, Clare Winnicott was ready to do something different. Before expanding on this, it is appropriate to consider the contribution that the child care courses had made. Jean Packman, writing about the impact of the six university child care courses, concluded, "The effect that those first few trained workers (and their tutors) had upon the new service was probably far greater than their numbers would imply. As pioneers, they were a strongly committed and sometimes exceptional breed" (Packman, 1975, p 11). These child care officers, most of them women, also played a leading role in establishing the Association of Child Care Officers (ACCO) in which John Stroud was also involved. The LSE courses certainly contributed their share of influential child care personnel.

In 1998, I published a book to mark the 50th anniversary of the 1948 Children Act. Much of it consisted of interviews with former children's officers, a number of whom had been taught by Clare Winnicott and paid tribute to her influence on them:

• Denis Allen was a pacifist who was jailed during the war. He maintained that his prison record then blocked his hopes of becoming a probation officer. It did not, however, stop him being accepted for the child care course at the LSE in 1951. He left the course convinced that child care officers needed to be part of a strong, professional body and he became an active member of ACCO. He also believed that the children's service needed trained staff and years later, as children's officer for East Sussex, he gave priority to winning resources for training both field and residential staff.

• Philip Hughes had been a radio officer on a ship escorting *The City of Benares* which was torpedoed despite the fact that it was full of evacuees on route to America. After the war, he joined the child care course at the LSE and subsequently rose to be deputy children's officer in Kent. With the LSE's training behind him, he was horrified "to find a low proportion of qualified staff" (Holman, 1998, p 43). He immediately strove to improve matters and won himself a reputation which helped him obtain the post of children's officer at the London Borough of Greenwich, where he again insisted on high standards.

• Margery Taylor had been a secretary during the war and afterwards was interviewed for a place on the social sciences course at the LSE. The interviewer started by saying that the last candidate was a WREN who had saved people from drowning, and what had she done? Margery had to confess that she could not even swim. She did win a place but later felt much more at home on the child care course. She was deeply impressed by Clare Winnicott, became the president of ACCO from 1962-63, and from 1965-74 she served as the director of training with the London Boroughs Training Committee. Clare's emphasis on training was reflected in Margery's words, "The thread that has run through the whole of my professional life is an awareness of the importance of training" (cited in Holman, 1998, p 8).

• Joan Beckett was a Cambridge graduate who went on the child care course where, as she put it, "I was well Winnicotted by Donald and Clare" (cited in Holman, 1998, p 25). Her friendship with the Winnicotts continued after her training when she worked in London and felt free to drop in on them. She later became the children's officer for the London Borough of Kensington and Chelsea.

No doubt other child care courses did similar work, although they were not as well known. The LSE child care course produced a generation of child care officers who were committed to deprived children, who wanted a professional service, and who believed in specialist training. Clare Winnicott was not the only capable member of staff on the course, but, as its leader, she was the one who held the course together and was the one most remembered by former students. What was it that so impressed them? The content of her lectures was highly relevant to students committed to child care practice and wanting a grasp of theory. But it was not just what she said, but the way she said it. I can still remember her presentations nearly 40 years later. She was small and enthusiastic. She moved around the room, full of vitality. She presented profound ideas in simple ways and illustrated complex material with vivid case examples from her own experience. Above all, she conveyed that child care officers were engaged in a tremendously important job and that it was within their powers to improve the lives of deprived children. Perhaps she taught with a social and psychological zeal which reflected the religious pulpit manner of her father. As Joan Beckett put it, "Clare Winnicott was remarkable, very pretty and intelligent, she became the kind of emblem of what we wanted to be" (cited in Holman, 1998, p 25). Daphne Statham, later to be a child care officer, lecturer and then director of the National Institute for Social Work, was uncomfortable with some LSE staff who, in tutorials, appeared to treat her as a client to be caseworked. She said, in an interview with me, that Clare was never like that, rather she was always straightforward, warm and interested. She concluded, "She was the kind of social worker I would not mind being like. She was a role model because she cared about people, because she communicated well and because she had 'street cred' – she had done the job. She stood up for children" (Statham, 2000, interview with author).

Director of child care studies

By the early 1960s, despite the efforts of the child care courses, the Children's Departments were still largely in the hands of professionally unqualified staff. In 1960 just 28% of child care officers in England and Wales and in 1963 less than 15% of residential staff were fully qualified. The shortage was partly due to the fact that the number of training courses remained small in numbers, but due more to the expansion of Children's Departments. Their tasks had increased following the 1963 Children and Young Persons Act which gave them a duty to undertake preventative work. In 1956, there had been just over 1,000 child care officers; by 1962 there were 1,500 with the numbers still climbing. Moreover, further legislation was anticipated which would give them greater involvement with young offenders.

Obtaining trained staff became the preoccupation of many children's officers, especially those in large urban complexes which were unattractive to staff. I have earlier written a history of the Manchester Children's Department which was under the leadership of an outstanding children's officer, Ian Brown. As a child, Brown himself had been in public care in the hands of the Poor Law. He was determined to provide something better for Manchester's children and perceived that this could best be done by trained child care officers who could provide both expertise and personal relationships. Unfortunately, he found enormous difficulties in recruiting qualified staff and, indeed, at times in recruiting any staff at all. In 1956, he reported to the children's committee of Manchester Children's Department that advertisements for child care officers had not produced a single application from a trained person. He persuaded the committee to adopt a policy of seconding existing staff to courses on the understanding that they would return to work for Manchester. The ploy enabled his department to have a few qualified staff but nowhere near enough to keep pace with the demands on them. The outcome was that staff were taking on ever larger caseloads which caused some to leave. In his annual report of 1962-63, Brown uncharacteristically chided the government. He wrote:

> While it was becoming increasingly obvious that additional steps needed to be taken to increase the supply of trained child care officers, there was little indication that the Home Office Central Training Council was

seized with the same sense of urgency as children's officers and local authorities, upon whom new burdens were rapidly falling. (cited in Holman, 1996, p 131)

A year later, Brown informed the councillors that the department was unable to fill 50% of its vacancies and that not one child care officer was professionally qualified.

Manchester's plight may well have been worse than most authorities, but it did reflect a national shortage of trained staff and a belief that the government should take action to ease the crisis. By the 1960s, the key child care training position was that of director of studies in the Children's Department of the Home Office. Its incumbent, Sybil Clement Brown, was due to retire in 1964 and members of the Association of Children's Officers (ACO) and ACCO began to lobby that Clare Winnicott should replace her. The government agreed and Clare was offered and accepted the post. It entailed a huge administrative and strategic leap. In Oxfordshire, she had overseen five hostels. At the LSE she had administered a very small child care course and then been a part-time member of the generic course. At the Home Office she was a civil servant responsible throughout England and Wales for the training of field, residential and managerial child care staff. She was 57, but retained the enthusiasm and drive of a much younger person. She also displayed an ability to make plans to address the crisis, the skill to win resources from the government, and the capacity to enable civil servants, child care associations and educational institutions to cooperate. Her plan was both to increase the output of existing courses and to initiate new emergency courses for child care officers, many of whom did not possess the educational qualifications for university courses. Brian Roycroft, as a children's officer who served on the training committee of ACO, recalled Clare attending a number of its meetings:

> She was very feminine and attractive. More important, she was very businesslike. She displayed tremendous skill in helping children's officers, most of whom were not trained themselves, to understand training. She had a clear objective, she wanted their backing for the new emergency courses but without compromising on standards. Some children's officers wanted to second staff to be rushed through courses and to return with a piece of paper saying they were trained. She was very tactful and I was full of admiration for her. She had a kind of banner over her head saying, 'I am not going to let standards drop just because

some children's officers want more trained people quickly'. (Roycroft, 1999, interview with author)

Joan Cooper, who was chief inspector at the Home Office Children's Department from 1965-71, later wrote of her:

> At the Home Office as director of child care studies from 1964 to 1971, when she received the OBE, Clare Winnicott led an able team of inspectors and supported by the then Central Training Council in Child Care, initiated and promoted an expanded training programme to meet the then demands of children's departments and voluntary organisations, and the projected extra 1,000 child care officers required for the 1969 Children and Young Persons Act. A partnership was promoted with the universities and colleges, together with emergency training for graduates and for older entrants, a national programme of in-service training for residential staff supplemented by BBC talks on child care to which Donald Winnicott contributed, refresher courses all over the country and the maintenance of the existing training programme. (Cooper, 1984)

Janie and George Thomas, both former child care officers, became lifelong friends of Clare Winnicott. Janie took over from Clare as a part-time lecturer at the LSE. She was also principal lecturer on the first emergency training course at the North West London Polytechnic. She wrote to me about the course, which had 100 students:

> All the students were over 35 years and each had to be sponsored by a local authority or voluntary agency where they did their second year placement. The practical work supervisors were all agency staff. It was the closest possible application of theory to practice. When Clare came to speak to the students they loved her. (Thomas, J., 1999, letter to author, 14 November)

Child care training took on an atmosphere of mission. Tutors and students shared an enthusiastic commitment to better the lives of deprived children. The number of child care officers in training rose from 174 in 1964, to 805 in 1971. The test was whether places such as Manchester benefited. They did. Ian Brown cooperated with the establishment of an emergency course at the Extra Mural Department of Manchester University and, by the end of the period, not only did Manchester Children's Department have a larger and full child care establishment, it also had one in which 33% were professionally qualified. The drastic improvement was due, as Ian Brown acknowledged, to the leadership of Clare Winnicott at the Home Office. The number of trained child care officers multiplied during this period, but many of the newcomers were very different from the graduates who had come through the one-year university courses. Keith Bilton, the first general secretary of ACCO, explained in an interview with me that he had gone straight from his Oxford degree to a social work course. He saw himself as typical of those from a middle-class background, with little experience of life, selected because of their academic achievements. He continued, "Clare Winnicott, by being the driving force behind the emergency two-year courses, drew in a large number of non-graduates, usually older, people with relevant experiences of life but with few intellectual qualifications" (Bilton, 2000, interview with author). In like manner, Daphne Statham, who headed-up one of the emergency courses, stated:

> She brought in people from a different class background. Some were women who had brought up children, some were people changing occupations having been teachers, nurses, in the forces, some had been unemployed and in poverty. They were different from young graduates. On the courses, they had two years to concentrate on child care and families and they left with the makings of competent child care officers. How different from today when child care gets taught in a few weeks. The important thing is that most of them tended to last at the job. (Statham, 2000, interview with author)

It should not be overlooked that Clare Winnicott was also concerned with training for residential staff. George Thomas had joined her team as an inspector. He wrote to me as follows:

> Clare had a flair as a team player. She kept on board, Home Office mandarins, local authority officials, the wider inspectorate and the varied and sometimes fiercely independent training institutions. Within this, she had a massive impact on residential child care training through preliminary child care courses for 16-18 year olds; in-service training modules ... the first residential options on field work courses; advanced courses for senior residential staff. (Thomas, G., 1999, letter to author, 14 November)

In a sense, the child care service was having to run just to keep up with itself. As fast as it turned out more child care staff, so the number of posts was increased, so that by 1970 it had risen to 3,741. The fact that by this date the proportion of qualified child care officers had grown to over a third thus represents a considerable advance. In Scotland, by contrast, efforts to improve matters resulted only in a fifth of child care workers being qualified. As my chapter on Barbara Kahan indicated earlier, similar achievements did not hold for the residential sector, partly because it did not retain qualified staff. Nonetheless, Clare Winnicott had succeeded in putting training at the forefront of child care. In 1970, Janie Thomas, then president of ACCO, toasted her with the words, "Clare Winnicott's name has become synonymous with training" (Thomas, 1970, p 9).

Building a child care profession

Clare Winnicott's contribution to child care is usually regarded as the establishment of training for child care officers, and rightly so. But training was a means to an end. Since her time in Oxfordshire, she was committed to creating the best possible service for deprived children. To her, this had three components, and she was active in each.

- First, the existence of a local authority agency devoted to deprived children and nothing else. She gave evidence to the Curtis Committee and rejoiced in the 1948 Children Act which created Children's Departments.
- Second, the availability of staff with the child care skills to understand the needs of children and to communicate with them, plus the commitment to stay with the children through thick and thin. These attributes, she believed, were most likely to be transmitted through specialist child care courses.
- Third, a profession of child care which would allow child care officers to support each other, which would advance skills, and which would lobby for the well-being of deprived children. Perhaps it is insufficiently recognised that Clare played a major part in building up ACCO. Adele Toye has written about ACCO's early days as follows:

> It was our tutor at LSE, Miss Clare Britton (later Mrs Winnicott), who gave us practical help as well as encouragement to tackle the work of forming an Association. At the end of the academic year in 1948, letters were exchanged between the various groups of students and a meeting of us all was arranged, during which we set up a Study Group to think about ways and means of creating a child care officers' association. Miss

Britton not only enlisted the help of Dr Winnicott, who provided the penniless Study Group with a free meeting-place, but she also persuaded several eminent members of other professional bodies to come to our meetings and give us the benefit of their experience. (Toye, 1970, pp 63-4)

One of the early issues was whether membership of ACCO should be restricted to professionally qualified child care officers. Clare was of the opinion that it should be open to all those employed as child care officers, whether qualified or not. Her reason appeared to be that to exclude the unqualified would be to exclude the great majority of practitioners and so make the association into a small and precious elite. By embracing all child care officers, the Association could broaden the skills base of its members. Not least, the larger the organisation, the greater its clout in terms of influencing outside bodies. This view prevailed and ACCO became the largest social work organisation whose views were taken seriously by government. Later it introduced a two-tier level of membership but the non-qualified staff were still able to participate fully. Keith Bilton points out that, subsequently, the experience of ACCO was influential in deciding the form of membership for the British Association of Social Workers (Bilton, 2000, interview with author).

From an initial membership of 12, ACCO grew to 2,589 members by 1969. All through these years, Clare and Donald gave their support, attended meetings and conferences and contributed articles to *ACCORD*. During its 21-year existence, ACCO gave honorary membership to only two people: Clare and Donald Winnicott. For Clare, it was important that child care officers had a strong professional body which could represent the interests of members, which could press for more training and which could lobby on behalf of deprived children. But it was more than that. Clare's concept of a professional was of a skilled, preferably trained, officer who was able and confident enough to make decisions about and be creative about the children and families for whom they were responsible. In a joint article with Donald, she wrote that "... it is the worker with originality and a live sense of responsibility that is needed ... the worker who loves to follow a rigid plan is unqualified for the task" (Winnicott and Britton, 1947).

But could creativity, originality and a live sense of responsibility survive in enormous bureaucracies? Could child care skills be retained as Children's Departments were amalgamated with other services into the new social services departments and social work departments in 1970-71? There is no doubt that Clare Winnicott had her doubts. She was the guest speaker at ACCO's final annual meeting in 1970, just before ACCO itself was incorporated into the British Association of Social Workers. As a civil servant of the government which was legislating the changes, she had to choose her words carefully. She praised ACCO on three fronts. First, for playing its part in "establishing a social work service within the local authority setting", a service which, she explained, was about personal relationships more than administrative procedures. Second, for "the development of the professional self-awareness and sense of identity of its members", an awareness and identity which was rooted in child care. Third, for its "vitality" which "springs from direct involvement with the work, with clients and their problems" so that members were not speaking about second-hand experiences (Winnicott, 1970, pp 74-6).

In what would now be called 'code', Clare Winnicott was expressing her fears that the creation of large social work super-departments would lead to administrative functions overshadowing social work ones, to the lessening of a sense of child care identity and skills, and to social work agencies in which many employees would be cut off from personal contact with clients. More directly, she admitted that she was saddened by the ending of the job title of 'child care officer' and added that she would be even sadder "if the concept of social work as a caring function were ever superseded" (Winnicott, 1970, p 77). She poured scorn on the idea that the needs of children were the same as those of older people and other client groupings. Obviously, she was worried that the new generic social workers – who were expected to deal with various kinds of clients – would lack the specialised skills to serve deprived children. She finished by challenging the new unified social work profession to somehow preserve "the immense differences between social work with clients in one kind of situation and another, and immense differences in social workers, which attract them to certain kinds of work and not to others" (Winnicott, 1970, p 78). Her words were hardly a ringing endorsement of the sweeping changes which were being made to social work. Brian Roycroft was present at her talk and said:

> The theme of her speech was 'don't lose what you've gained in child care skills'. At the time I was very disappointed because we were all interested in becoming social service directors. There were a number of significant people then who were either very far-seeing or very backward looking because they were not happy about the Seebohm concept and warned that what we had gained in child care could be lost. (Roycroft, 1999, interview with author)

So, in 1970, the Children's Departments for which Clare had campaigned were abolished. The ACCO to which she had been a kind of social midwife was dissolved. So, too, was the Children's Branch of the Home Office while the Central Training Council in Child Care was amalgamated into the Central Council for Education and Training in Social Work. Clare left with a great sense of loss. Worse was to follow. On 25 January 1971, Donald suffered a fatal coronary at their home. Their marriage had been an extremely happy one. David Donnison remembers that, on one occasion, Donald saw a passing flower cart and spent £50 on its whole load of peonies – Clare's favourite flower – and spread them all over the house. David also revealed that Clare had told him that her only regret was that she had never had a baby by Donald. Not surprisingly, after Donald's death, Clare experienced a depression that led her to re-enter psychoanalytic treatment under Dr Lois Munro, a psychiatrist whom she found very helpful.

Somewhat to her surprise, Clare was invited back to the LSE as head of the Social Work Department and, as such, leader of the applied social studies course. It was not what she had expected. The student world had changed dramatically since her previous days at the LSE. Many students were protesting about societal injustices, were involved in local community action and, within their colleges, were questioning what was taught and, in some cases, participating in sit-ins and demanding more say in the way courses were constructed and evaluated. Many social work students were frequently asking what older social workers were doing to challenge poverty and they were particularly critical of casework and psycho-dynamic approaches which they regarded as a means of social control. Many of them were at one with Adrian Sinfield who, in a Fabian Society pamphlet stated that many social workers "seem to see little relevance in the problems of inequality" and were persuading people to tolerate the intolerable (Sinfield, 1969, pp 12-13). Keith Bilton explained, "Some of her ideas were anathema to radical social workers. In some of her articles, she seems to regard delinquency as explicable purely in psychological terms and with no reference to factors like poverty" (Bilton, 2000, interview with author). It was all so different from the days when admiring child care students had hung on her every word. Janie Thomas pointed out to me that Clare continued to have students who admired her at the LSE but added, "It was not a happy time for her and in many quarters her beliefs were losing their influence" (Thomas, J., 1999, letter to author, 14 November).

Before long Clare retired. In 1974 she was diagnosed as suffering from a melanoma on her foot which failed to respond to innumerable operations.

Disillusioned with what was happening in the field of social work, she devoted her twilight years to editing Donald's writings, to practising as a psychoanalyst, and maintaining her contacts with a wide circle of friends and family, particularly with her niece, Alison. David Donnison had not seen her for some years but got to know her again during this time. He said, "My marriage broke up in 1979 and I moved to Glasgow. It was a very difficult and painful time. I found my way back to Clare to talk to her, not so much as a patient, I wasn't seeking counselling, but I found it a healing experience" (Donnison, 2000, interview with author). Clare's sister, Liz, moved in to share her London home but in 1979 she was killed by a car as she was crossing the road. Clare's brother, Karl, died in 1983 while her other brother, Jimmy, outlived her and died in 1994. Clare's last years were ones of increasing infirmity, but she insisted on getting out and going to social occasions. She died on 15 April 1984, at the age of 77. Her many friends felt a deep and genuine sense of loss. As David Donnison remarked, "I felt quite bereft when she died" (Donnison, 2000, interview).

Janie Thomas was with Clare when she died. Clare had a great capacity for sustaining friendships and it is therefore appropriate to record what Janie Thomas wrote to me about her:

> From the mid 60s right through until her death, we were good friends. She was such fun to be with. She was one of those rare people with whom one could have 'interior to interior' discussions – a precious gift of friendship in a world where so much conversation is 'external'. You could always be your true self with Clare and relate on an equal footing as friends, despite her brilliance. (Thomas, J., 1999, letter to author, 14 November)

Clare Winnicott is certainly remembered by friends, but she is rarely quoted in today's social work literature. This is partly because she wrote very little. During and just after the war, she wrote a number of articles or chapters (often in conjunction with Donald) about the work of the hostels. Subsequently she wrote a few articles, the best of which were gathered together in *Child care and social work* (Winnicott, 1964). But she wrote no major social work text. Daphne Statham said, "She wrote well. She had a wonderful mind and was able to combine theory and practice. I can never understand why she wrote so little" (Statham, 2000, interview author). Daphne wonders if Donald absorbed 'too much' of her life. Certainly Clare was overshadowed by her husband. He was one of Britain's foremost child psychiatrists whose books had enormous sales. Brian Roycroft said, "Donald had the international reputation, you didn't look right in your car unless you had one of his books on the floor. But she was the clearest and sharpest thinker of the two. I went to a number of parties at their house and she seemed to mother him" (Roycroft, 1999, interview with author). If she did mother him, did boost his career, then it was her choice. She devoted much of her time to him, always making sure that his dinner was ready on time, and watching his health very closely. After his death, she made sure that nearly all of his unpublished writings were published. Clare Winnicott thus chose to promote Donald's writings rather than her own.

One by-product of Clare Winnicott's close identification with everything that her husband said and wrote was that some students and social workers dismissed her as wanting to turn social workers into mini-psychiatrists or psychotherapists. This was far from the truth. Certainly, she wanted child care officers to be competent in what she called casework, that is, in making a close, personal yet professional relationship with children (and their carers) in order to help them understand and deal with their feelings and behaviour. Yet she also taught quite explicitly that child care officers helped children by changing their environments. Indeed, she stated that "The child's primary need is not for a casework relationship but for an environment which can provide for him and within which he can be cared for successfully" (Winnicott, 1964, p 11). By environment, she was referring to the care provided by parents, foster parents or residential staff. A child care officer could change the environment by enabling the parents to function more adequately, by providing suitable foster parents or by settling children with residential staff capable of giving them guidance and affection. One of the main differences between psychoanalysts and child care officers was that the former rarely attempted to change clients' environments while the latter were consistently trying to improve them. It is true, however, that Clare was less comfortable with the practice of community work in which workers might improve local conditions, initiate youth amenities, campaign for reduced rents and so on in order to improve the social circumstances of children and parents. Her discomfort was surprising given her background in youth work. As a young lecturer, I once asked her at a public meeting whether tutors should be equipping child care officers to work with communities as well as families. Her response was that it was outside the sphere of social work.

Despite her small published output, Clare Winnicott, mainly through her talks and lectures, was a leading figure in the 1950s and 1960s in establishing just what was the core of child care social work. Her main themes can be briefly enumerated.

First, in her Oxfordshire days, she insisted that children in care could not be treated as though they had no parents. She revealed that she was "given no idea of the whereabouts of the parents of children in care because they were thought to be irrelevant" (cited in Packman, 1975, p 137). She then spent enormous time and effort in tracking down relatives. Thereafter, she taught students that they should attempt to avoid taking children away from their parents and, if the children did enter care, then they should seek to reunite them. While in care, they should try to maintain contact between children and parents and enable children to face up to their sense of rejection and anger at having to leave their families.

Second, she strove to show that children in care were more than administrative units. Clare's early career overlapped with the last years of the Poor Law when reception into public care depended on whether an application fitted into certain rules. Children's feelings and emotional needs were not at that time taken into account. Even in the initial years of some Children's Departments, applications from parents were processed by clerks. Clare Winnicott challenged such inhumane treatment by emphasising the enormous impact on children of being parted from their parents. She added that the very moment of uprooting from one environment to another was psychologically crucial to a child and explained "that a skilled child care officer is needed to see that what a child clings to in the past is brought with him and accepted in the new environment" (Britton, 1954, p 179). She maintained that a toy, an old blanket, or anything that was part of a child's past, was so important that the child should be encouraged to take it with him. This was the very opposite of administrative tidiness which might prefer to leave old possessions behind. She was not dismissive of the administrative setting, however. Indeed, in one of her best known articles, 'Casework and agency function', she showed that child care officers' objectives and powers were defined by the nature of their agency (Winnicott, 1964). Rather she taught that administrative action, rules and procedures were not sufficient to help deprived children.

So what was considered to be a child care officer's basic tool? According to Clare, it was the priority given to the professional relationship between social workers and clients. Although Clare had welcomed the Curtis Report's emphasis on the need for personal relationships within child care services, she was careful to point out that staff could not give all of their personality and time to children. She therefore preferred to talk about the professional relationship within which child care officers related closely and warmly with children (and others), but in ways defined and limited by the purposes and duties placed on them by their agency. Within this relationship she saw them as doing the following:

- Understanding as much as possible the child's past experiences. Some of this knowledge could be found in written form in files and reports, some from speaking with other significant people in the children's lives, and some directly from the child.
- Conveying to the child "the feeling that somebody sees his point of view and understands and can tolerate his feelings, whatever they are" (Winnicott, 1964, p 16).
- Acting as the essence of reliability in a child's life so that they knew where to find their child care officer and knew that their attitudes and values would be constant.
- Being able to communicate with the children. Sometimes this was expressed in friendly chat, in jokes and laughter, in enjoying an outing or trip together, in discussing school, work and play. At other times, it was more indirect, with the child care officer reaching the child by what was called 'a third object': whereby something else might be going on, like watching the television, which allowed the child to continue at one level until they were ready to go to a deeper level. With this concept, Jacobs gives Clare the credit for having "introduced a particularly useful tool in communicating with children" (Jacobs, 1995, p 137). In addition, communication entailed dealing with the child's deepest fears, angers and emotions. Clare took care to point out the dangers of dealing with feelings. Nonetheless, she insisted that children should be given the opportunity to look at the trauma, the pain, the sense of loss, the bewilderment, associated with leaving their families and being moved from one place to another. She believed that child care officers most needed training in the sphere of communicating, learning how to grieve with children, how to help them express their anger, how to explain to them what was happening. She felt that they had to find "the alive bit" in the child, the issue they most wanted to deal with (Britton, 1954, p 179). Obviously, such communication took child care officers into emotive areas. But Clare Winnicott did not want them to wallow in depression. She believed that the relief of pain helped the children to grow. She explained:

> Having reached the child we try to look at his world with him, and to help him to sort out his feelings about it; to face the painful things and to discover the good things. Then we try to consolidate the positive

things in the child himself and in his world, and to help him make the most of his life. (Winnicott, 1964, p 57)

Nearly 40 years on, I can still recall Clare Winnicott's message and words in one lecture on childhood deprivation. She said, "The important thing is how the child deals with it". She pointed to some well-known political figures who had succeeded in life despite deprived upbringings. Other victims never recovered. Her point was that adverse effects were not irreversible and that a skilled and communicative child care officer could help victims to positive outcomes.

In order to maximise the effectiveness of the professional relationship, Clare Winnicott considered it important that child care officers understood themselves. She did not say that they had to be psychoanalysed before they could help others – far from it. She said, "The most fundamental thing we have to know about is the strength of our own feelings about the sufferings of children" (Winnicott, 1964, p 43). She meant that staff could be so angry about the neglect and ill-treatment of children that they adopted a rescue motive of taking children away from parents, thinking the emotional slate would then be wiped clean, and letting the children start anew with other adults. Yet the children still had feelings for those parents and the emotional slate could never be wiped clean. Again, child care officers might be so horrified at what had happened to children that they veered away from discussing it. The officers had to understand when it was *their* feelings and not the needs of children which were shaping their actions.

Does child care social work need the likes of Clare Winnicott today? Three people, all well qualified to judge, believe that it does.

- Daphne Statham asserts that standards of child care practice are now much more varied than in the days of the Children's Departments. She said, "Some practice is the best there has ever been. But we have lost a lot. I am appalled at the lack of knowledge about child care, about the effects on children of loss and being moved around. I am appalled that some children seemed to be treated more like numbers than individuals. We need to recover Clare's capacity to see the whole child and to see them as individuals" (Statham, 2000, interview with author).
- Keith Bilton stated, "We still need her ideas today. She had a wonderful grasp of the relationship between practical help and the more interpersonal aspects of social work. The union of these two is the

essence of social work" (Bilton, 2000, interview with author). He believes that this kind of social work has declined.

- Joel Kanter, who has probably studied her writings more closely than anyone else, highlights her capacity to train students to be sensitive to the needs and difficulties of deprived children and to be able to communicate with them. He asserts that "these methods for communicating with children are rarely taught to social workers today on either side of the Atlantic" and regrets that "her personal approach to children and other persons in need is in conflict with the increasing bureaucratisation and mechanisation of social work practice" (Kanter, undated, pp 76, 85).

Clare Winnicott's working life stretched from the 1930s to the 1980s. As a young youth worker, she saw and grieved over the poverty of children at the very time Eleanor Rathbone was making the case for family allowances. After the war, she rejoiced that the welfare state had alleviated some poverty, but she never ignored the fact that many families still had unmet practical needs. Just as the war-time evacuation of children was a turning point for many reformers, so it was for Clare Winnicott. Her experience in hostels for evacuees, along with meeting Donald, convinced her that deprived children required help via relationships with skilled children's workers. It was also during this period that she observed that children in the hostels needed knowledge about and contact with their natural parents and siblings. John Stroud may well have been influenced by her writings as he became a practitioner who always sought to reunite children separated from their families. Further, Clare reasoned that skilled child care practice was most likely to flourish in local authority departments which specialised in deprived children. She was thus at one with Lady Allen in the campaign which led to the establishment of Children's Departments.

Many of the new Children's Departments were blessed with children's officers with the kind of drive and vision most clearly seen in Barbara Kahan. In addition, the departments required trained child care officers to undertake the day-to-day contacts with children. Clare Winnicott, more than any other individual, promoted training. Initially at the LSE and then at the Home Office, she taught and then organised courses which equipped and inspired a multitude of staff. She was indeed the personification of child care training. Simultaneously, she understood that the new occupation of 'child care officer' would be strengthened by its own professional body. With the likes of John Stroud, she played a part in building ACCO.

There were others who led stimulating child care courses. There were others who freely gave of their time and effort to ACCO. But she was the children's champion who defined, described and taught the skills with which staff could help children who were traumatised and damaged by experiences of loss and separation. Even today her writings and insights have not been surpassed. She worried that the amalgamation of Children's Departments into social services departments would lead to a decline in these specialist child care skills. Barbara Kahan, in fact, was one who believed that this did happen.

Clare Winnicott concentrated mainly on children separated from their parents, whether poor or not. And at the LSE she was a colleague of a young lecturer who was to focus on the plight of all poor children, Peter Townsend.

SIX

Peter Townsend, 1928-2009

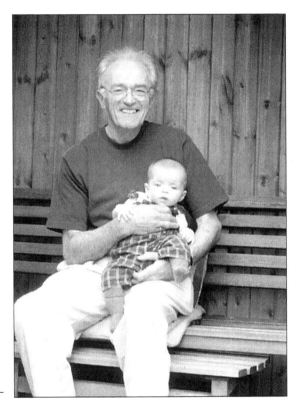

Photograph of Peter
Townsend and his
grandson, kindly sup-
plied by Peter

One of Peter Townsend's earliest memories is of playing cricket with the comedian Arthur Askey. They met while Peter's mother was performing in a seaside revue. Peter was to become Britain's leading poverty researcher and campaigner against child poverty.

Childhood

Peter's parents were living in Middlesbrough when he was born in April 1928. The marriage soon broke up and Peter saw little of his father for years. By the age of three, Peter was living in London where his mother was pursuing her career as a singer and stage performer. As Peter recorded in an interview with Professor Paul Thompson (now lodged in the Essex University Archives), "We had a very chequered existence because some weeks she was very much in work, and other weeks she wasn't" (Thompson, 1999, p 2). His mother's intermittent earnings meant that Peter sometimes experienced the hard side of life. From an upstairs flat in Pimlico with the cooker on the landing, they moved to an attic flat in Belsize Park and then to a basement flat in the same district.

Sometimes Peter's mother took him on her tours. On one occasion, during the war, she was performing in Blackpool and lodging in a boarding house. Years later Peter wrote about this experience, that he noticed how people were shocked "by the poverty of the evacuees. In the early part of the war the upheavals of evacuation caused many people to understand for the first time how the other half lived, and what the years of unemployment had wrought. Here were two nations confronted" (Townsend, 1973, p 1). Back home, as a teenager, he also took his turn as a fire-watcher, enjoyed the sense of fellowship with others and observed the readiness of ordinary people to make sacrifices for others.

Although his mother took him on some tours, during most of them he stayed at home with his grandmother. In an interview with me, Peter spoke movingly about his mother. He said:

> Because she was on the stage and being the breadwinner, she was sometimes an aloof figure. Here was this very attractive figure on the platform and I looked at her with wonder from a distance. There were many warm occasions and I remember nestling in her lap and listening to music hall on a Saturday evening. But that kind of affectionate intimacy is not my predominant memory of childhood.

> She dried up on stage in her early forties and retreated into a phase of alcoholism which was augmented, unfortunately, by an association with a man with the same predilections. As a young man, I was strangely unable to help her. I was in the army and then university and so physically away from her. She wanted me to succeed but, because of her lack of education, she wasn't familiar with what I was going through so there was a distance – which often happens between working-class children who go to university and their parents. (Townsend, 2000, interview with author)

Peter's maternal grandmother accompanied them to London and she was the one who cared for him on a daily basis. He said, "My grandmother was the key figure in my life. She took me to school and I returned at lunchtime for dinner. She was the person I was in touch with everyday" (Townsend, 2000, interview). A warm, dependable, motherly person, she not only gave Peter love and affection but also – by her helpfulness to others – became to him a model of a caring and accepting person. In addition, Peter recalls that "her accounts of poverty in Middlesbrough were dramatic, especially the wooden coffins of young infants on her shelf in the kitchen. She had to take in washing to make ends meet because she was a lone parent whose husband had disappeared. Almost unconsciously, I became aware of poverty" (Townsend, 2000, interview).

Peter went to a local authority elementary school where his teacher, Miss Sard, spotted and encouraged his talents. In 1939, aged 11, he passed the scholarship to the prestigious University College School, one of the few schools to remain open in London during the war-time blitz. Here, Peter said, "I was influenced by the headmaster, partly because I had not been close to a man" (Townsend, 2000, interview). The headmaster was C.S. Walton, who encouraged pupils to question established thought; for instance, he set exams where everything was done to distract the pupils, like the sudden playing of loud music. Peter explained that "it established the point that everything, even exams, is socially constructed. I saw that wealth and the way it is shared out is politically and socially constructed" (Townsend, 2000, interview). Meanwhile, Peter not only shone academically, but also captained the school at both cricket and rugby. As school captain, he took the courageous step, with the headmaster's agreement, of abolishing the school's cadet corp. At the age of 16, he became an ardent church-goer, although this tailed off after a couple of years.

A year later, in 1945, Peter rejoiced in the landslide victory of the Labour Party. Looking back at that event he wrote:

> A transformation had taken place. In the Britain of 1945 it seems possible to detect the two human impulses which, as I understand it, are necessary to any Socialist society…. There was an attitude of trust, tolerance, generosity, goodwill – call it what you like – towards others; a pervasive faith in human nature. Then there was a prevailing mood of self-denial, a readiness to share the good things in life and to see that others got the same privileges as oneself. (Townsend, 1973, pp 2-3)

Clearly, Peter Townsend was politicised as a young man. The process continued when he went into the army for two years' national service. He declined the opportunity to be an officer and remembers that his interest in politics increased, "I suppose partly because of the mixture of classes that I encountered in the Nissen huts" (Townsend, 2000, interview).

In 1948, Peter took up a place at St John's College, Cambridge, where he studied philosophy and social anthropology. He commented to Paul Thompson that the anthropological research approach was to prove important to his later studies. He was drawn by "the idea that you did not do things in an aloof way, you didn't send out teams of juniors to collect your data and you sat at home in comfortable situations ... and wrote your reports but you actually lived, you got engaged with that society" (Thompson, 1999, p 23).

His relationship with Cambridge was a love–hate one. He loved the facilities for learning and research, but he hated the elitism and the class distinctions which made it difficult for students from working-class backgrounds to fit in. He also disliked the social differences between town and gown and, while editor of the undergraduate newspaper, he wrote an article on that theme. In 1952, his writing experiences helped him obtain a post as a research assistant at an institution called Political and Economic Planning (PEP).

Research apprenticeship

Peter's first task at PEP was to write a pamphlet called *Poverty: Ten years after Beveridge* (Townsend, 1952). In it he argued that the levels of government benefits had been set far too low. He also challenged the findings of the third Rowntree poverty study of York which had asserted that poverty had virtually disappeared, with only 1.66% of the population being poor (Rowntree and Lavers, 1951). The 24-year-old Townsend was thus criticising the famous Seebohm Rowntree and co-author of the report, Commander G. Lavers. Before the pamphlet was published, Lavers angrily protested to PEP and insisted on a confrontation with Townsend. Peter's measured arguments against the methodology of the York study won the day and the publication of the pamphlet went ahead.

His next assignment was a study of the effect of unemployment on former cotton workers in Lancashire. After consulting officials, he started interviewing unemployed people. His first interview was with a woman who, with her husband, had been earning £12 a week as weavers. Their social security benefits totalled £3.14s for themselves and two children.

Peter was profoundly moved both by the sufferings of these families and by their strengths in adversity. It reaffirmed his conviction that a researcher had to rely as much on direct communication with those in poverty as on contacts with academic experts and textbooks.

He was only at PEP for two years, but this was an important time when Peter formulated some of the themes that were to remain with him for the rest of his life. He challenged the subsistence notion of poverty which was inherent in both official benefit scales and in much poverty research. He drew on actual interviews with unemployed citizens to argue that these existing scales did not provide for an adequate standard of living. He started to assert that any concept of poverty had to be seen in the context of the incomes and lifestyles of the rest of society.

In 1954, Peter accepted a post as a research officer at the Institute for Community Studies which had been founded in East London by Michael Young. His particular study concerned the pattern of life among older people in the area. Through interviews, he discovered an enormous diversity of experience where some enjoyed the enrichment of constant contact with many relatives while others were lonely and isolated. Clearly, the existence of family, particularly the extended family, was the major source of support for older people. In addition, Peter identified the importance of mutuality, the fact that the "happiest and most secure relationships ... seem to be those in which all kinds of services are exchanged, as when the old grandmother cooks the meals and cares for the children, and her daughter does the shopping and cleaning and works part-time outside the home. One-sided dependence is disliked and the ability to give, to be of use to others, to do one's share and to be independent, is venerated" (Townsend, 1973, p 17). The book based on the research, entitled *The family life of old people*, was met with good reviews and ran to several reprints (Townsend, 1957). The quality of the study no doubt contributed to Peter's appointment to the London School of Economics and Political Science (LSE) in 1957 as a research fellow and subsequently as a lecturer.

The London School of Economics

The Department of Social Administration at the LSE was probably the foremost centre for the study of social policy in Britain. David Donnison included Townsend when he referred to "the finest team of researchers in that field to be found anywhere in the world" (Donnison, 1982, p 18). Two of the team were to be particularly important to Peter. One was the head of department, Professor Richard Titmuss. Townsend admired him as someone who, without any academic qualifications, had worked his way to the top through his sheer intellectual brilliance. Although Titmuss was an emotionally reserved man, Peter looked on him as a father figure and stated that "he was an adviser to me about what to make of my life, and I suppose – more in terms of the example he set – I gained enormously from that.... The other thing I gained from him was his ability to turn over a question, and look at it from different perspectives" (cited in Thompson, 1999, p 65).

Peter was even closer to Brian Abel-Smith, an aristocrat, 27th in line to the throne, who had become a socialist while at the famous public school, Winchester College, and who was already at the LSE when Peter arrived. But they had met earlier. Peter explained to me, "We met in London in 1952 when we had this parallel impulse to write about poverty. He was more theoretical about equality. He was very angry but more from a kind of spirit of the enlightenment. It was the force of the intellect rather than of experience or empirical knowledge. Mine was founded in the back streets of Nelson and Colne, meeting unemployed men and their families" (Townsend, 2000, interview with author). In later years, Peter had some disagreements with both Titmuss and Abel-Smith over the issue of means testing: Peter being firmly opposed to it in principle and practice. Nonetheless, they remained great influences on his research and beliefs.

Peter's initial appointment at the LSE was as a research fellow, for which he had a research grant from the Nuffield Foundation to make a national study of residential institutions for older people. His book, *The last refuge*, published in 1962, revealed an enormous variety of provision ranging from small private homes with four residents to huge institutions, often based in the old workhouses, with over a thousand occupants (Townsend, 1962a). One personal lesson for Peter was that the Labour government certainly had not created the new Jerusalem (meaning the new, better society as used in the title of the book by Andrew Davies [1992] *To build a new Jerusalem: The Labour movement from the 1880s to 1990s*).

Little will be written here about Peter's continuing interest in older people and other specific vulnerable or disadvantaged groups such as disabled people, those with mental illness and people from ethnic minority groups. The focus here is on his studies of poverty as a whole. Encouraged by his promotion to the post of lecturer and by the support he received from Titmuss and Abel-Smith, he further extended his investigations of, and writings about, poverty. In 1962, he published a paper entitled 'The meaning of poverty' in which he drew much of his thought together (Townsend,

1962b). He started by questioning the assumption that the welfare state had abolished poverty. While acknowledging that legislation had introduced a range of benefits for unemployed, sick and older citizens, Townsend went beyond most other social commentators by attacking the benefit levels. He pointed out that they derived from Seebohm Rowntree's investigations, which stretched back to 1900, in which it was assumed that an adequate income was enough to secure the 'physical efficiency' of individuals. He criticised the way in which Rowntree had made his calculations and argued that, to survive on the Rowntree rates, families would have to be experts in cooking, budgeting and knowing where the cheapest food was available. He pointed out that Rowntree subsequently allowed for more than physical efficiency by conceding that recipients should have enough to buy items such as newspapers. The issue then became what kind of other needs should be met, should they include holidays and leisure? Further, Townsend explained that social needs change with, for instance, the possession of a radio becoming almost a necessity. In short, as he put it, "Poverty is a dynamic not a static concept". He then went further and asserted that this subsistence notion of poverty had to be replaced by a relative one. He concluded by writing, "Our standpoint, then, should be that those individuals and families are in poverty whose resources, over time, fall seriously short of the resources commanded by the average individual or family in the community in which they live, whether that community is a local, national or international one" (Townsend, 1962b).

In the midst of all his research, teaching, writing and public speaking, Peter was also a family man. He met Ruth Pearce in a London park when she landed a snowball on his ear. She was the daughter of the president of the British Dental Association, who was later knighted. Ruth and Peter married in 1949, while he was at Cambridge. Once Peter secured employment in London, they moved to a terraced house in Hampstead where Ruth devoted much of her time to looking after their children, Matthew (born in 1952), Adam (1953), Christian (1957) and Ben (1962). Peter regretted that often he was not home until after 7 pm, but nonetheless, he was an interested, affectionate and participative father who particularly enjoyed making up stories to tell the boys. Weekends allowed him more scope to take them to the park where he taught them cricket, football and athletics. The Townsends also mixed with their neighbours and Peter stated, "I remember keenly, Ruth looking after one lovely woman living locally, for some weeks and months, in her terminal illness" (cited in Thompson, 1999, p 220).

The poor and the poorest

Among Peter's multiple activities was a major study of poverty which he completed in cooperation with Brian Abel-Smith. They did not receive a large research grant to facilitate interviewing a cross-section of the people. Instead, they hit on the idea of using existing government statistics. Following the war, the government had undertaken periodic household expenditure surveys which contained information on the incomes of a large sample of the population. They obtained permission from the Ministry of Labour to examine the original questionnaires and to use the relevant statistics for the years 1953-54 and 1960. They would then not only have figures whose accuracy could hardly be doubted, but also they would be able to assess change over a six-year period.

The government surveys provided information on incomes but they did not define poverty. Townsend and Abel-Smith took the prevailing rates paid by the National Assistance Board (NAB) as their baseline and then assessed how many people had incomes below this level, how many were on the level and how many were 40% above it. The latter, which they called the 140% level, was chosen because many social security claimants received regular additions such as exceptional needs payments which took them above the minimum rate.

The results were surprising. They showed that for 1953-54 an estimated 600,000 people had incomes below the base level, while overall 4 million (7.8% of the whole population) were living at less than the 140% level. For 1960, the figures had grown to 2 million and 7.4 million respectively. Among the findings which caused most comment was that 2.2 million children were among those below the 140% line (with 600,000 below the basic NAB rates). Clearly the problem of low income was not one confined to older people. Further, the numbers not only included those dependent on benefits, but also some in full-time work. When the study was published in December 1965, it was entitled *The poor and the poorest* (Abel-Smith and Townsend, 1965). Noticeably, the authors did not use the word 'poverty' in the title but the content of the book made the case that extensive poverty still existed in Britain and that even the introduction of family allowances had not actually abolished child poverty.

Abel-Smith and Townsend had hoped that their findings would prompt the government to take action, but they were to be disappointed. As Peter said to me, "I went to 10 Downing Street with Brian to see Harold Wilson and he made dutiful noises about the importance of the recognition of child poverty. We thought it would have been much more effective but nothing much transpired" (Townsend, 2000, interview). Nonetheless, the study did have significant outcomes and Professor Rodney Lowe considers it "a major turning point in British post-war social policy" (Lowe, 1995). For a start, it overthrew the conventional wisdom that poverty had been virtually abolished and would eventually wither away. Further, it succeeded in shifting the discussion and study of poverty away from a subsistence notion of how much money was required to allow people to survive, to one in which the government's own scale rates were used as an indication of how many people were in need. Peter did not claim that this was a scientific measure of poverty, but it did mean that the problem was beginning to be recognised and produced the hope that new research could establish the nature and extent of poverty.

Not least, the study had an impact on social work. Other chapters in this book indicate how Children's Departments led to the development of the occupation of child care officers who regarded their clients much more humanely than pre-war officials had. Nonetheless, many still regarded poverty as the result of inadequate personal functioning. As a student on the child care course at the LSE, I received no systematic teaching about the extent and explanations of poverty. Then, as a young child care officer, I recall reading *The poor and the poorest* and believing that the explanation of poverty rested less in individual deficiencies and more in the structural failings of the state. Casework could do little to change the mechanisms which distributed resources. However, like a number of other social workers, I realised that we could equip ourselves with welfare rights skills to ensure that our clients received their full dues from the social security system.

Lastly, as Rodney Lowe puts it, the study "provided the stimulus for the creation of the CPAG [Child Poverty Action Group], one of the first and most prominent of the expert pressure groups which the 1960s established as a permanent feature of British welfare politics" (Lowe, 1995).

The Child Poverty Action Group

Among those who contributed to the formation of the Child Poverty Action Group (CPAG), Harriett Wilson was one of the most prominent. Born in Germany, she had settled in Britain in the 1930s and, during the war, experienced some hardship as a lone parent. After taking a degree at the LSE, she worked among socially deprived families in Cardiff and wrote an influential book *Delinquency and child neglect* which dwelt on the adverse effects of poverty on family life (Wilson, 1962).

Harriett was a Quaker and met regularly with others to discuss poverty.

In 1964, the Labour Party had been returned to power and, in 1965, Harriett arranged a meeting at Toynbee Hall, London to consider the failure of the new government to improve family allowances, which had not been increased since 1956. About 20 people, including members of the Family Service Units (FSUs) who had close contacts with the poorest people in Britain, gathered to hear Brian Abel-Smith present some of the results of the forthcoming *The poor and the poorest*. Peter Townsend subsequently joined the meetings and CPAG was launched with Fred Philp of the FSU as its first chair.

On 23 December 1965, one day after the publication of *The poor and the poorest*, CPAG submitted a memorandum to the Prime Minister. It drew heavily on the Abel-Smith and Townsend study but reinforced it with research which showed that poverty was related to early mortality and under-achievement at school. It concluded, "It is necessary to find a way to increase the income of the poorer families with dependent children, both when the head of the household is employed and unemployed. We believe that this can best be done by increasing family allowances or by making some modification of the child tax allowances that will benefit poor families" (CPAG, 1965, para 15). In August 1966, Tony Lynes was appointed as the group's full-time secretary and the CPAG journal, *Poverty*, was launched. CPAG was now into its first phase as an organisation in which the emphasis was put on attempting to show that poverty was a real and important issue. It also started to address some of the claims of right-wing writers that state welfare provisions were harmful to society.

In 1969, Frank Field replaced Tony Lynes as the director of CPAG, while Peter was elected as its chair. Frank was a talented Labour councillor and former lecturer. He was clearly set on a political career and later became an MP and government minister. Field and Townsend were a formidable, although not always harmonious duo, who took the group into its second phase in which it contended that government was not acting to counter family poverty. Soon the group was arguing that, under the Labour government, a sharp increase in National Insurance contributions, increasing unemployment and rising prices were making life worse for the poorest members of society. It called on the government to increase family allowances and to claw back the money by raising taxes on standard rate taxpayers.

On 27 January 1970, Field and Townsend were summoned to meet the Minister for Social Services, Richard Crossman. Interestingly, Peter faced his friend Brian Abel-Smith across the table, who had accepted a position as a government advisor. Peter had declined suggestions to take up a similar post, partly because of his dislike of the government's immigration policy. But he graciously acknowledges that Brian was probably much more adept at the role. He said, "Probably because of his aristocratic roots and because the civil service is so dependent upon an Oxbridge background, he was an acceptable figure and therefore a great influence in the corridors of power" (Townsend, 2000, interview).

Frank Field has described the meeting in graphic terms, writing that the minister, Crossman, "banged the table, he shouted, and he mocked. There was an endless machine-gunning of sarcastic jokes to which the civil servants responded as if part of a mediaeval court". Field was uncertain how to react, but he added, "Peter Townsend quietly argued back against the torrent of abuse" (Field, 1982, pp 32-3).

Following the meeting, CPAG released the memorandum it had presented to Richard Crossman. It provoked controversy, as the press seized on it to headline the claim that the poor had got poorer under a Labour government. Ministers reacted with some fury. In April 1970, Ann Shearer reported in *The Guardian* on a lengthy speech made by David Ennals, a minister at the Department of Health and Social Security:

> ... [he] unleashed a speech which very nearly accused the group of lying, and of betraying its friends by feeding ammunition to the Opposition. At the same time, he attempted to buy it back with offers of closer co-operation and a hint that the increased family allowances that it wants may be on the way. (Shearer, 1970)

Several papers ran the same story and also reported on a radio interview with Peter. *The Birmingham Post* quoted him as saying, "Mr Ennals resorted to mud-slinging. The group works in two rooms in an attic. It is a shoe-string organisation and here we have the whole weight of the government brought to try to crush this organisation because it is saying facts" (*The Birmingham Post*, 1970).

For some months during this period, Frank Field was ill so Peter undertook much of the CPAG work. This coincided with an intensive amount of pressure at Essex University to which Peter had moved. Frank Field later praised Peter's contribution:

> ... it is relevant to stress the key importance of Peter Townsend's role in the transition from the period when Tony Lynes was running the Group to the ten years when I was responsible for its development ... it is

doubtful if the campaign would have been taken so seriously as it was without his presence as chairman of the Group. (Field, 1982, p 34)

Labour lost the 1970 election and some blame was directed at CPAG for its 'The poor get poorer under Labour' campaign. Peter rejects this accusation. With regard to the campaign, he said to me, "It was a calculated move to cause the government to make up its mind long before the likely election. Wilson called an early election and thereby made our recent criticisms an almost inevitable aspect of discussion at the election" (Townsend, 2000, interview). Despite the acrimony promoted by the attacks on the Labour government, the outcomes were not all negative for CPAG. As Frank Field concluded, "Poverty had been moved back towards the centre of the political stage and was being discussed widely in Parliament and the media" (Field, 1982, pp 34-5). In 1970, the Conservative shadow chancellor, Iain MacLeod, met CPAG and committed the next Conservative government to an increase in family allowances. Unfortunately, MacLeod died later that year and the pledge was never kept.

During the ensuing years, Peter and Frank continued to work closely together. Peter says of Frank, "He proved to be an extraordinarily versatile campaigner with a political twist" (Thompson, 1999, p 200). Frank's setting up of the Low Pay Unit was seen as particularly important. The unit was organisationally separate from CPAG but united by Frank's leadership and it served to demonstrate that low pay as well as low benefits was a part of poverty. While highlighting Frank's contribution, Peter is eager to explain that CPAG as a whole was involved. He recorded that CPAG "sparked Frank into doing things which the rest of the group wanted and which were creative and which were influential" (Thompson, 1999, p 200). In like manner, Frank acknowledges CPAG's debt to Peter Townsend. In an interview with me, Frank said, "He is a great figure. His standing was of immense importance to CPAG. He – and the treasurer Garry Runciman – projected an image which made it hard for people to disregard". He adds that CPAG also gave Peter "a public platform to express his views", a platform which made for greater coverage than from university lectures and academic books (Field, 2000, interview with author). Later the two men differed sharply over some issues, particularly when Frank advocated the sale of council houses. But their mutual respect continues to this day.

Frank left CPAG in 1979, when he was elected to the House of Commons. CPAG then entered what Peter Townsend sees as its third phase of consolidation. Under the able directorships of Ruth Lister, Fran Bennett and Sally Witcher, it established its role of educating people both about the existence of poverty and about the fact that governments were failing to address the problem. CPAG grew in terms of numbers of staff and publications and in its role as comprising the leading welfare rights experts in Britain. Much of this occurred while Ruth Lister was at the helm. Now a university professor, she commented to me on Peter's time as chair as follows, "He was very committed and gave a good lead. He was not the lead person as in the early days when CPAG was very small. He allowed staff to have scope and was not breathing down our necks. If you wanted advice, he was there. He encouraged us to think widely, such as about poverty in its international context, whereas we were just concerned with the next Bill before Parliament. He is one of the few people who have got more radical as he has grown older and he would probably have liked us to be more radical" (Lister, 1999, interview).

Peter considers that, for some of the 1980s, CPAG "was not quite sure where to move during the Thatcher years. Some think a much more strident, campaigning phase might have been more successful. Attempting to persuade the Thatcher government to make a few concessions was possibly not the right course" (Townsend, 2000, interview). At the same time, he is pleased that CPAG had not followed the pattern whereby "organisations tend to become less radical as they grow older, they grow well organised and efficient but also bureaucratic and institutionalised. Organisations where the leaders are trying to cultivate the award of a knighthood or OBE tend to succumb to the blandishments of government. CPAG has avoided this" (Townsend, 2000, interview).

In 1989, Peter retired as chair, partly because of the demands of his intensive involvement with the Disability Alliance. He was made president of the group and continues in that role to this day. When he attends meetings in CPAG's large and modern building in White Lion Street (which cost £1.43 million), with its rows of publications and its extensive training programmes, he must find it hard to believe that all this grew from a shoe-string organisation which met in rented rooms with no staff. Of course, CPAG has its limitations and both unfriendly and friendly critics. The unfriendly critics, often from the New Right, regard it as part of the poverty industry which has a vested interest in obtaining grants to study and campaign about poverty. Of the friendly critics, David Donnison is typical; he is another former LSE professor and one-time chair of the Supplementary Benefits Commission. Donnison said, at a meeting which discussed the history of the CPAG, "It was highly metropolitan, very London-centred, and professional both in the best sense of that term and in the elitist sense, developed by people who were marvellous at talking with politicians, to civil servants in the Reform Club or wherever they met, but much less likely to be mobilising the poor themselves and getting them on to platforms or working with grass-roots groups"(Lowe and Nicholson, 1995). Frank Field, while not contesting this view, is convinced that CPAG reached and influenced poor people. He wrote, "Slowly, more and more poor people are seeing their poverty less as a sign of personal failure, and more as a result of the actions of governments and an electorate which supports these governments"(Field, 1982, p 74). The criticism that CPAG spoke for, and not with, poor people has been a consistent one and other organisations have sprung up in an attempt to be vehicles for poor people. However, it must be said that the group welcomes and works alongside these agencies. What is not in doubt is that CPAG can list many achievements.

CPAG is Britain's foremost poverty lobby. Before the 1960s, Britain did not possess an influential poverty group. By the late 1960s, CPAG had, as Field points out, "a decisive influence on policy" (Field, 1982, p 23). It is true, as Field acknowledges, that the Prime Minister of that period, Harold Wilson, did not give it "a single line mention" in his memoirs (Field, 1982, p 24). Nonetheless, the fact that CPAG was blamed by some government ministers for Labour's electoral defeat and the fact that senior Conservative politicians approached the group indicate that it had become a force to be reckoned with. CPAG can take credit for putting poverty back on the political agenda. And, during the Thatcher years, when the government was not keen on discussing poverty, CPAG, as Ruth Lister said, "was a thorn in the side of the Conservatives and opposed many of its attacks on welfare" (Lister, 1999, interview). Peter Townsend sums up that CPAG "is now probably recognised as an international force, highly efficient, and one which politicians of all kinds have to take seriously" (Townsend, 2000, interview).

By keeping poverty in the eye of governments, the media and the public at large, CPAG has put particular emphasis on the value of family allowances – child benefit as it is now called. Eleanor Rathbone rightly saw benefits as a major means of alleviating child poverty without imparting stigma. Established by the 1945 Family Allowance Act, their continuance has not always been assured. As Peter Townsend remembered:

> In the 1960s, family allowances were very much under threat. There were surveys which showed numbers of older women who said, 'We managed without them, why should mothers have them now?' CPAG corrected misconceptions about family allowances. When he became chancellor, Nigel Lawson wanted to abolish them. He couldn't because

he was hedged around by 'wet' Conservatives who prevented it. This is significant if you consider the other means taken in the 1980s to wreck and dismantle the welfare state. (Townsend, 2000, interview)

CPAG has constantly and successfully argued for the retention of this benefit as a universal benefit paid to mothers and also, with less success, argued for it to be increased in line with the growth of real earnings.

As well as being a campaigning and lobbying movement, CPAG also established its Citizen's Rights Office. Today this is *the* source of welfare rights information whether it be for claimants, for their advisors or for journalists. It also advocates on behalf of individuals and takes up relevant poverty issues with the courts. Its handbooks are the welfare bibles for all involved in matters of social security and low pay. Ruth Lister said, "It gave a great impetus to welfare rights activity which has now spread so that many local authorities see it as their function" (Lister, 1999, interview).

Despite its growth, CPAG has maintained its commitment and enthusiasm. Its staff include long-serving people like Sue Brighouse and Beth Lakhani, who retain the same values as the founders of CPAG. Its director is now Martin Barnes, of whom Peter Townsend and others have high hopes.

CPAG has achieved much and a lot of its growth has been due to Peter Townsend. *The poor and the poorest* was one of the main factors which drove concerned individuals to start the group. As chair in the 1960s and early 1970s, he cooperated with Frank both in writing CPAG's material and campaigning on many platforms. During the 1980s and 1990s, his own standing stood CPAG in good stead. David Bull joined the Executive Committee of CPAG in 1967 and succeeded Peter as its chair in 1989. David Bull is, therefore, well placed to make an assessment of Peter's contribution, and did so in a letter to me. He wrote that Peter's "huge expertise was notable for its generosity, modesty and its inspiration". He explained that, first, "he was so generous in the amount of time he unstintingly gave to CPAG – whether in attending meetings of the Executive Committee and many a sub-committee of which he was but an ex-officio member or in meticulous attention to the laboured drafts of those of us who lacked his startling ability to write so coherently at first draft". Second, "this was all done with extreme modesty: everybody had his or her say; he delegated trustingly and was just another member of the team. You only ever saw him distance himself from the team on social occasions when he so often seemed incapable of small talk – which is odd when you consider how natural he was in the company of children.

It wasn't that he was socially aloof with adults: he'd just quietly slip into the background or do the washing up". Third, inspiration:"How blessed we were at CPAG to have access to the finest macro-mind I ever associated with ... he was capable, in a committee meeting, of teasing out just about any issue that was raised. This could mean that he spoke more often from the Chair than you'd expect and the meetings might run on, but I can't imagine that many committees have been so educated, even on a Friday evening, by such genius from the Chair" (Bull, 2000, letter to author, 1 March). To many people, CPAG and Peter Townsend are usually spoken of in the same breath.

University of Essex

In 1963, at the academically youthful age of 35, Peter was appointed Professor of Sociology at the University of Essex. He never regarded the post as the means of a salary to enable him just to do research and have his work published. He set about building up the teaching of social policy at undergraduate and postgraduate levels and, in a short space of time, the department gained a national reputation. He also entered fully into wider university affairs in this new university. He objected to the existence of a senior common room which separated staff from students at mealtimes. He believed that the integration of staff and students "still gives Essex some of the flavour of its mixing ..." (Thompson, 1999, p 180). The case for separate facilities, he argued, rested on the assumption that staff "deserved special treatment" (Thompson, 1999, p 180) and this went against his fundamental belief in equality. This belief also gave him some understanding of the student protests which loomed large in the University of Essex in 1968. He remembers almost fondly "when we had General Assemblies and a thousand people attended them in a new university, and that thousand people included the porters and the cleaners as well as secretaries and professors" (cited in Thompson, 1999, p 180).

From 1975 to 1978, Peter served as University Pro Vice Chancellor. He recorded, "I had a function outside the Department. And I'm proud of holding rents down (for student accommodation) ... and probably more important, establishing the Day Nursery. I don't think this would have happened without me hammering away at it" (cited in Thompson, 1999, p 189).

After 19 years at Essex, Peter moved to a chair at the University of Bristol where, once again, he set about building up the teaching and research of social policy. It was not an altogether happy move. He commented that "the experience at Essex was one of novelty and expansion. The experience at Bristol was one of decline.... There was a long University struggle about cuts, cuts and more cuts" (cited in Thompson, 1999, p 192). David Bull, who was also a colleague of Peter's at Bristol, wrote, "His dogged pursuit of his research and writing made him a colleague to be proud of but not always to work with, in the day-to-day demands of departmental administration. His irritation with these demands, and with the different ways in which some of us expected to meet them, made him a lot less exciting to work with full-time than to collaborate with at CPAG" (Bull, 2000, letter to author, 1 March). Bristol was difficult for Peter but there were positive features and he recorded, "But at Bristol, I think more successfully than I'd managed at Essex, I did personally ... teach a course in each year at every level – first year, second year, third year, and at Mastership, and PhDs, throughout the period and that kind of thing gave me inner satisfaction" (cited in Thompson, 1999, p 193). Another positive development at the University of Bristol was that Peter was able to develop his interest in the connection between ill-health and poverty, a subject of which more will be said later.

One of the reasons that Peter moved to Bristol was to be nearer to Jean Corston. His marriage to Ruth had broken up while he was at Essex. It had been decided that Ruth and the children would stay in London, partly because the boys were starting at comprehensive schools there. Peter therefore commuted 60 miles to the University of Essex at Colchester. Eventually he took lodgings at the university. The enforced separation, the demands of a new job and Peter's continuing heavy involvement with CPAG, contributed to the break up with Ruth in 1974. Peter began a relationship with a colleague at the university, Joy Skegg, who he married, and in 1976 their daughter, Lucy, was born in Colchester Hospital. Peter recorded, "it was like a second chance at being a father ... for the first four years of Lucy's life, I did as much in her upbringing, physically, as Joy did ... we shared the upbringing of Lucy until, in 1980, I met Jean, and really appreciated that I had made quite a big mistake in the 1970s, and that I'd now met the person who meant most to me in my entire experience" (cited in Thompson, 1999, p 238).

Peter met Jean Corston at the 1980 Labour Party Conference. He recalled, "I think that it's one of those extraordinary occasions that not many people have the luck to experience, of love at first sight" (cited in Thompson, 1999, p 242). Jean had left school at the age of 16 and worked for trades unions. She and Peter married in 1985 and she went to the LSE to read law and qualified as a barrister, as by this time her own children were grown up. Soon after, she was elected a Labour MP. Their relationship has brought Peter much happiness but it entailed, for the early years, the agony of his separation from Lucy. He stated, "Joy didn't want to speak to Jean and it was a terrible job to try to obtain access. And when I did obtain access, it was through a very stiff, uncomprehending and unsympathetic welfare officer, through the courts, who gave grudging terms of access, so that effectively, I got to coming up to London to collect Lucy, going to Bristol and taking her back to London from Bristol" (Townsend, 2000, interview).

Poverty in the United Kingdom

It is difficult to convey the extent of Peter Townsend's research, writing, lobbying and campaigning in one chapter. In the mid-1980s, he undertook a new survey of London life and labour, with special reference to poverty. Not all of the study was written up but among the material published was an article that attracted a lot of attention, written with Paul Corrigan and Ute Kowarzik, called *Poverty and labour in London* and published by the Low Pay Unit (Townsend et al, 1987). By way of further example, Peter also acted as a consultant to studies abroad. One was in Kenya where Peter discovered that he was being paid "the white colonialist's rate by UNESCO [United Nations Educational, Scientific and Cultural Organization]" (Thompson, 1999, p 153) while his three Kenyan colleagues received far less. Peter requested that they all be paid the same and, when this was refused, he resigned. The sheer amount and variety of Peter's input can be seen in a booklet issued on his retirement from the University of Bristol after 18 years. It lists his publications and papers for the years 1948-94 and stretches to 44 pages, which is about 440 items.

Here attention must be drawn to his famous study and survey of poverty completed while he was still at the University of Essex and funded by the Joseph Rowntree Memorial Trust. The book *Poverty in the United Kingdom* contains an in-depth analysis of the meaning and nature of poverty and leads to the definition that "people can be said to be in poverty when they lack the resources to obtain the types of diet, participate in the activities and have the living conditions and amenities which are customary, or at least widely encouraged or approved, in the societies to which they belong" (Townsend, 1979, p 31). The study was based on a survey undertaken in 1968-69 in which nearly 7,000 people were interviewed. The interpretation and write-up of the material involved a team of researchers whom Peter admired and who later went on to successful academic careers. They included Dennis Marsden, Adrian Sinfield, Alan

Walker and John Veit Wilson. From a book of 1,200 pages, only a few of the main findings can be presented here. Most importantly, Townsend used three measures of poverty. The first was the state standard, that is, those living below, on, or just above the levels of Supplementary Benefit. He recorded that 11.86 million people (21% of the population) were in this position. The second was the relative income standard consisting of those with less than 50% of average income: 16.10 million people (29%) were poor by this measure. Third was the deprivation standard in which he devised a measure that took account of imputed income from capital and services. Accordingly, 12.56 million (22%) were in poverty.

Interestingly children and older people were the largest groups affected by poverty, closely followed by disabled people. Substantial poverty was found among the employed as well as the unemployed. Noticeably, means-tested benefits were shown to have severe limitations with, for instance, around 40% of those eligible failing to take up Supplementary Benefit and free school meals. Turning to inequality, the study showed that 5% of the population owned 45% of net assets and that, when income was combined with wealth in a measure of resources, the top 5% had an advantage nearly 10 times that of the bottom 10%.

In the face of such poverty, Peter identified six themes for countering it, namely the abolition of excessive wealth, the abolition of excessive income, the introduction of an equitable income structure, abolition of unemployment, reorganisation of employment and the reorganisation of community services.

The responses to the study were both numerous and mixed, and have been documented by the Qualitative Data Archival Resource Centre at the University of Essex, from which the following are a selection; first, unfavourable reviews:

> Masquerading as a moralist, Peter Townsend is in fact nothing more nor less than a political propagandist, confusing ethics with ideology. (Peregrine Worsthorne, *Sunday Telegraph*)

> The incredible magnitude of his figures ... suggests either that he is entirely deficient in common sense or, more feasibly, that he is determined that the poor should continue to exist and multiply in order to vindicate his own political beliefs. (Leader in the *Daily Telegraph*)

> A deformed picture.... The absurdity is, the more generous you are to the poor, on his kind of assumption, the more they will multiply.... A

mountain of nonsense and distortion.... This is not a work of scholarship, in my opinion (Lord Harris of High Cross, *Now*)

"I reject Professor Townsend and all his works.... It is no more than common sense to acknowledge that as a nation becomes more prosperous, so the numbers in poverty are reduced. The Townsend approach, so beloved of the left, simply feeds the politics of envy...." (Speech by Patrick Jenkin, Secretary of State for Social Services)

There were also many appreciative reviews, for example:

In this bible for the poverty lobby, he draws together all the information about poverty, inequality and the distribution of resources in the United Kingdom.... What he and his colleagues have in fact achieved over the last 15 years is something far more important than the rediscovery of poverty. They have redefined it. Townsend's rejection of absolutist measures of poverty and his commitment to an egalitarian, relative definition amounts to a new moral standard and a rejection of the approach adopted by his predecessors – William Beveridge, the Webbs and Seebohm Rowntree.... It is an outstanding achievement. (Professor David Donnison, Chair of the Supplementary Benefits Commission, *Glasgow Herald*)

This is the largest Penguin Book ever produced. It may prove to be one of the most useful and possibly the most influential. (*Local Government Chronicle*)

To conduct and bring to completion a project of this scale is not only a feat of intellectual persistence, but an entrepreneurial accomplishment. (Peter Oppenheimer, *The Listener*)

Peter took the criticisms in his stride. He said to me, "By that time I was aware that if you believed what you were doing was right and if it was built on a sound scientific basis, then you stood for it. You can't just retreat, you have to accept and meet criticisms. I was quite exhilarated that it made a public impression and I spoke at meetings all over the country. I have tried to mobilise public opinion. It didn't have an impact on government and the Conservatives rejected poverty as a worthwhile problem with one of its ministers, John Moore, on record as saying that poverty didn't exist. Monetarism was taking over and any suggestions about redistribution were seen as beside the point and impractical" (Townsend, 2000, interview with author).

Not surprisingly, *Poverty in the United Kingdom* made little impression on the Thatcherite governments. But, even more than *The poor and the poorest*, it stimulated debate about poverty: its extent, its nature, its causes and the means to tackle it. Since its publication, no study of similar magnitude has appeared. Certainly, Peter Townsend was applying moral values to the judgements he made. He did – and does – believe in a more equal society. But he recognised and articulated those values. His critics who clung to the old minimalist or absolute meanings of poverty failed to recognise that their judgements were also shaped by values. Twenty years later, Peter still holds to his belief that relative poverty is both wrong and unnecessary. The indications are that his views are winning ground. Today he says that *Poverty in the United Kingdom* is the book of which he is the most proud.

Poor health, poverty and inequality

From the days he went out interviewing unemployed people in Lancashire, Peter believed that poor citizens were more vulnerable to ill-health than their more affluent counterparts. In 1977, the Labour government set up a Working Group on Inequalities in Health under the chair of Sir Douglas Black, formerly chief scientist at the Department of Health. Peter was pleased to be appointed as one of the three other members (the other two were J.N. Morris and Cyril Smith). The report was ready by 1980 and demonstrated not only a clear link between poor health and inequality, but also that health inequalities were widening, largely because material inequalities were increasing. Among its many recommendations, the Black Report (as it became known) recommended higher levels of welfare benefits and a more equal distribution of income (DHSS, 1980). However, by 1980, the Conservatives were in office and the Secretary of State for Social Services, Patrick Jenkin, arranged that a mere 260 copies of the report be made available – and on a bank holiday weekend. In a dismissive foreword, Jenkin declared that the expenditure involved in the report's recommendations was unrealistic even if they would be effective. Peter's response was, in conjunction with Nick Davidson, to publish a popular version of the report as a Pelican book (Townsend and Davidson, 1982). It soon went to two re-printings and is still available. The Black Report was, in Peter's view, of great significance. He stated, "It was the first report to show that inequalities in health were growing, that even if absolute health, in some senses, was improving, that relatively the gains were being experienced more among the upper income groups more rapidly ... it was still quite evident that material deprivation accounted for more than half the difference between rich and poor in the inequalities of death...." (cited in Thompson, 1999, pp 142-3).

In 1997, the newly elected Labour government established an Independent Inquiry to examine health inequalities. Chaired by Sir Donald Acheson, it confirmed the link between material inequalities and a range of illnesses, diseases and conditions. Prominent among its 39 recommendations was that government should "further reduce income inequalities and improve the living standards of households in receipt of social security benefits" (DoH, 1998a, p 203). Although the New Labour government followed up some of the Inquiry's less controversial and less expensive suggestions, it ignored its emphasis on reducing income inequalities.

Meanwhile, Peter was pleased that the interest in health at the University of Bristol had come to a head in a centre named in his honour, the Townsend Centre for International Poverty Research. It produced the most up-to-date statistics, ranked according to parliamentary constituencies, in its book *The widening gap* (Shaw et al, 1999). The six most unhealthy constituencies were shown to be in Glasgow. I live in one of them, Ballieston, and among its figures are the following findings:

• 54% of its households contained children in poverty compared with 13% for the healthiest constituencies;
• its infant mortality rate was 80.4 per 10,000 compared with 43.2 per 10,000 in the healthiest constituencies;
• 41% of its adult men were unemployed or permanently sick compared with 11% in the healthiest constituencies.

These figures are examples of the huge health differences between different areas.

Nationally, it showed that the infant mortality rate in the poorest families was 70% higher than in those in the highest socio-economic class and that those in the lowest class were four times more likely to die in an accident. Moreover, the gaps throughout Britain were widening with, for instance, the life expectancy rate gap between men in social class I and social class V rising to 9.5 years. The findings were a further confirmation of Peter's argument that health inequalities were both wide and widening.

Involvement with the Labour Party

Despite his dispute with the Labour Party in 1970, Peter Townsend has remained a long-time member and supporter. From 1954 until the late 1980s, he served on various committees of the party. He does not consider them altogether useful exercises and recorded, "I remember frequent occasions when Barbara Castle was in the chair of the Labour Party Social Policy Committee or Social Security Committee … where she just wanted to get the meeting over with quickly, and carry on with what she'd been doing" (cited in Thompson, 1999, pp 198-9). That has not, however, prevented him in the last few years from becoming a staunch supporter of Barbara over pensions. At least, as he pointed out to me, he did produce papers for the party, particularly on disability, community care and superannuation. He believes that some of his proposals, for example on community care and the attendance allowance, were later taken on board but "I cannot easily identify specific results and I played no part in the run-up to the election of 1997" (Townsend, 2000, interview).

What does he think of the achievements of New Labour? He acknowledges that the increases in child benefit, small improvements in Income Support rates and the introduction of the Working Families' Tax Credit at least indicate that New Labour – unlike the previous Conservative governments – wants to alleviate poverty. However, in his interview with me, he made the following points:

- Child benefit increases were long overdue, and are still not up to their earlier value in relation to earnings.
- Financial help has been directed mainly at working families. This does not mean that all workers are getting a proper wage but it does mean that the incomes of non-workers have been neglected.
- The government has taken no steps to determine just what is an adequate income for all families.
- Above all, Peter regrets that the government is not committed to the basic socialist aim of reducing material inequality. He explains that, although between 1994-95 and 1997-98 the weekly incomes of the bottom 20% of households rose, they did so much less than those in the top 20%. He fears that inequality may actually widen under New Labour.

So what can be done to address poverty and gross inequality? Peter insists that an initial step is to show that change is possible. He points out that it was actions taken by the Conservative governments of 1979-97 which multiplied poverty and inequality, that if they had not undermined social security benefits then the poorest 20% of the population would today have about £5 billion or 20% more in aggregate disposable income and that the ratio between them and the richest 20% would be 1:5 instead of 1:9. It follows, he argues, that present governments could take action to reverse the trends. He adds that greater financial equality is compatible with economic growth and cites Finland, the Netherlands and Japan as economies where greater equality has accompanied national prosperity.

So if his aims are accepted as desirable and feasible, what specific steps does he envisage? First, that standard child benefit for each child be increased to 5.5% of average gross male earnings. Second, that an infant care allowance and additional age-related benefits for children be introduced. Third, there should be an expansion of the services of free milk for the under-fives, free school meals for all children and improved maternity grants for mothers. Fourth, the level of disability benefits at every age should be raised.

The objection to such proposals is still that which Patrick Jenkin levelled against the recommendations of the Black Report: that the country cannot afford them. Yet the costs of its recommendations (which include the four specified above) updated to 1996, would come to £12.5 billion, 1.7% of the GDP, or less than a tenth of current expenditure on social security. Where would this come from? Peter wants the personal taxation system to be reconstituted both to put some constraint on high incomes and also to raise money for public use. He also recommends the so-called Tobin tax of 0.25% on every transaction within the financial markets, a tax which would not harm companies but which would raise billions of pounds (Townsend, 2000, interview).

Townsend in his seventies

This chapter has outlined the remarkable and long career of Peter Townsend. What is he like today, now that he is into his seventies? He says of his marriage, "I'd never stop if I was trying to recount my indebtedness to Jean, my wife! I'm just one of those very lucky people who found someone relatively late in life, who met every kind of need that one has for male/female relationships" (cited in Thompson, 1999, p 214). He remains in positive contact with his four adult sons. Lucy has completed a degree at Manchester University and has continued to stay with Peter and Jean on many weekends.

He has not retired to tend his garden, although growing vegetables is a hobby. He did return to the LSE, where he has a personal chair. He said to me,

> The nature of my activities has shifted more emphatically towards the international scene. My chair here is in international social policy which involves not only social security matters but also the World Bank and international policy. One of my more important experiences was going to Georgia in the former Soviet Union where I encountered the colossal problem of the impoverishment, the starvation, of a third of its citizens. It once had a sophisticated system of social security and pensions which were utterly destroyed by an inflation rate of 2000% in the early 90s. Then the IMF and the World Bank recommended a crash programme of privatisation of its social services. They even had to wind up bread subsidies. I argued that there had to be basic services for a minimum income. There is still a need to recognise that poverty is an international problem. Social polarisation is destabilising and is the world's most fundamental problem at the moment. We are being self-destructive by not getting greater equality in terms of relationships and resources. The three richest men now have the same resources as the poorest 41 countries. This is a crazy world and something has to change. There is a deepening social hierarchy which divides the top from the bottom. (Townsend, 2000, interview with author)

In 1993, Peter published *The international analysis of poverty* (Townsend, 1993). He then contributed to a major study of the measurement of poverty within a European context. With David Gordon he edited *Breadline Europe* which appeared in early 2001. The book's starting point is that poverty is "more than having a relatively low income" and that measuring poverty as "half average household income" – the measure favoured by many European governments – tells little about what is a decent or acceptable income (Gordon and Townsend, 2000, p 17). The book distinguishes between two kinds of poverty, both of which can be measured: absolute poverty, which means "being so poor that you are deprived of basic human needs" and lack the resources to ensure adequate diet, housing, heating, clothing, sanitation, health services and education: then there is overall poverty which entails lacking the resources to live in a safe environment, to keep up with family and social duties and relationships, "to do all the things expected of you in your work", to feel part of your community, and to meet essential transport costs (Gordon et al, 2000, pp 87-8).

Jonathan Bradshaw draws together 14 measures of poverty in use in Europe. He points out that, "It is striking that the UK has the highest child-poverty rates but not the highest individual or household poverty rates". Putting the measures together and ranking them reveals that the UK is the poorest among 12 European countries (Bradshaw, 2000, p 228).

Peter Townsend: a summary

Peter Townsend's career has been so long and his activities so manifold that it is difficult both to summarise his achievements and also to convey something of his character. As already indicated, he has had his critics. Right-wing members of the Conservative Party have attempted to pour scorn on his claims that poverty is a major and multiplying problem, and Peter has just endured the attacks. As he said, "I've learnt to resist discouragement" (Townsend, 2000, interview).

Another criticism, given his identification with disadvantaged people and with the Labour Party, concerned his academic objectivity. As Rodney Lowe put it, "Was such party political commitment compatible with independent academic research?" (Lowe, 1995). Interestingly, the criticism was rarely levelled against academics who opposed him. Peter's answer has always been that his research methods are rigorous and open to the tests of scientific method and that he has the right of every other citizen to campaign about their findings.

One person who knows Peter well, but did not wish to be identified, said, "He can be very warm and supportive. But he did have bust-ups with people and [can] sometimes be rather thoughtless and this tended to come when he was doing too much". Having met him on a number of occasions, I know that he is friendly, interested and charming. But he will not give ground in discussions and is not reluctant to express his disagreements. He worked very closely with Richard Titmuss and Frank Field, yet he later had arguments with them over issues of policy which, for a while, soured their relationships. David Bull points out that, within CPAG, "he tended to see his view (as expressed in print) as the party-line" and this led to strong disagreements with CPAG members who publicly differed with him (Bull, 2000, letter to author, 1 March). Peter himself says that his two broken marriages caused unhappiness for the adults and the children involved, and he also acknowledges that some of his friends were critical of his behaviour. Like us all, he has his critics and his failings, but they should not detract from the enormous strengths of his character and achievements.

Peter's commitment to combating poverty is part of his very being, but it is not the whole of his life. He has family relationships, a circle of good friends, he enjoys music and reading and still follows the sports at which he excelled, namely athletics, rugby and cricket. Nonetheless, as he himself wrote, "My first serious piece of research was into poverty and the subject has remained my central preoccupation" (Townsend, 1973, p xiii). Since 1952, not a year has gone by without him publishing something on the subject of poverty. He was a founder member of both CPAG and the Disability Alliance and was the chair of both organisations for over 25 years. His commitment to opposing poverty comes before that to the Labour Party. Following the defeat of the party after its administration of 1964-70, he critically analysed its failure to deal with poverty and wrote, "Loyalty is a precious commodity and yet loyalty to Party can sometimes conflict with loyalty to socialist principles" (Townsend, 1972, p 5). His attacks on the party for not addressing the problem of poverty continue to this day. They do not endear him to the political establishment and he will never get a 'cosy' job at Westminster or Millbank. But for him the war against poverty comes before personal advancement.

Peter's commitment and also his perseverance are linked with his integrity. Having committed himself, as a young man, to socialism and to the socialist objective of equality, he has held on to them both as a politician and as an individual. He insists that the key question to be asked of any Labour government is, "How far had the social policies ... reduced inequality?" (Townsend, 1972, p 6). He has little sympathy for those who 'water down' their beliefs once they attain ministerial office. He has even less for those pseudo-socialists for whom "equality of sacrifice" is a principle which applies to others but not to oneself (Townsend, 1973, p 21). Peter himself has never been a champagne socialist; he has always refused a tenth of his income, and has scornfully dismissed any hints that he should go to the House of Lords. Instead he draws on George Orwell who "taught that socialism was a code of conduct to live by and not an uneasy compromise with vice" (Townsend, 1973, p 4).

Mention of the great writer, George Orwell, brings up another feature of Townsend – the sheer quality of his writings. Professor Ruth Lister commented, "He is not a brilliant lecturer. He is a brilliant writer" (Lister, 1999, interview). Frank Field admires his former colleague's capacity to present a finished article in beautiful English without going through numerous drafts. He is, says Field, "the George Orwell of the social services" (Field, 2000, interview).

Peter's commitment, his political integrity, his writings, are all an attack on poverty. His greatest contribution has been both to change the perception of poverty and to consistently keep it before politicians, the public and the media. Poverty is no longer regarded as 'just enough' to maintain physical efficiency. John Moore and those who deny the existence of poverty now make little public impact. A relative concept, which views poor people within the framework of the rest of society, is accepted even if their income is still too distant from the affluent. Much of the credit for this must go to Peter Townsend. So, too, the reforms which are being made by New Labour owe much to his detailed arguments and his consistent proclamation of socialist values.

Lastly, I have been struck by one other feature of Peter's character, namely, his nearness to disadvantaged people. The fashionable chattering classes may express sympathy for the poor and may approve of social reforms but often they get no nearer to them than hiring these people as servants to clean their homes and to tend their gardens. Some academics write books on poverty while maintaining a distance from them. Perhaps because his own upbringing brought him into contact with a wide range of people, Peter seems comfortable with those for whom he campaigns. Indeed, he has always insisted that he should maintain contact whether by interviews or other means. While collecting material for his study of older people, he took short-term jobs as an attendant in two institutions. In one – a former Public Assistance building – he was responsible for bathing the men, a task which he tried to do in such a way as respected their dignity. These experiences gave him some insight into what it was like to be one of hundreds of men who knew that they would spend the rest of their days in crowded, unsavoury environments.

I witnessed Peter's approach more recently. When the Conservative government refused to set up a commission on poverty, Channel 4 Television established its own in 1995. With Peter as its chair, its brief was to define and describe poverty, to explain its causes, and to make recommendations as to how it could be combated. It led to a TV documentary and a published report (Townsend et al, 1996). Among the deprived areas visited by the team was the one where I live, Easterhouse in Glasgow, where the commission met residents and walked the streets. One of the members of the commission, a well-known public figure, held views and attitudes which irritated Peter beyond measure and the sparks flew between them.

Simultaneously, Peter soon engaged with local people, put them at their ease, listened to them, took them seriously and made notes of what they were saying. Afterwards, a number commented on his warmth and concern. Only a handful met him in Easterhouse. All over Britain there are millions of poor people, most of whom may not know it, but in Peter they have a lifelong friend.

*   *   *   *

This book has been about six great children's champions. The first, Eleanor Rathbone, led the campaign to establish family allowances which have alleviated child poverty. The next four, Marjory Allen, Barbara Kahan, John Stroud and Clare Winnicott, were the foremost figures in creating Children's Departments and in improving the quality of care for deprived children. The sixth, Peter Townsend, is clearly in the Eleanor Rathbone mold of combating poverty. Yet, more than she, he also identified with and tried to improve social work services. His famous study *The last refuge* revealed the failings of institutional care for older people (Townsend, 1962a). He has had a lifelong commitment to the well-being of disabled people. His interest in the personal social services was reflected in a book *The fifth social service* (Townsend et al, 1970). One of his consistent themes is "the value of care at home rather than in an institution. Most children taken into care by local authorities and by voluntary societies, old people in need of care and attention, and young and old in mental and general hospitals may be better cared for in ordinary private homes within the environment or a normal or substitute family" (Townsend, 1973, p 20). Like Eleanor Rathbone, Townsend sees family allowances as one means whereby low-income parents can be enabled to retain the care of their children. Like Marjory Allen, Barbara Kahan, John Stroud and Clare Winnicott, he also understands that money is not always sufficient and that skilled child care social workers are required both to prevent families breaking down and also to deal with the emotional wounds of children who do enter public care. These six people certainly deserve the title of 'champions for children'.

Bob Holman, 1936-:
A child care participant living
through the changes

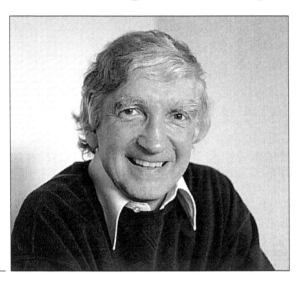

Photograph of Bob
Holman, reluctantly
supplied by Bob

It has long been my intention to record the lives and achievements of notable children's champions. When I submitted my proposal, I was delighted with the publisher's enthusiasm. However, there was a sting in the tail. They wanted a final chapter about myself. Their reasoning was that this would bring the story up to date and would touch on 'child care in the community' which was not a major theme of the six great figures. I am no child care champ, more a child care chump. But I have been close to most of the figures in this book and I am one of many whose own work has been shaped by their example. Further, I have had a personal life and a social work career which has coincided with the major social welfare events in Britain in the last 50 years of the 20th century. So, in this penultimate chapter, I will write, reluctantly, about my participation in these changes.

Participating in the evacuation (1939-45)

My paternal grandfather and grandmother came from rural Essex to urban Barking to look for work, and my grandfather found a job as a bricklayer. The early years of the 20th century were not easy for manual workers and in 1904 he became unemployed. There was no state unemployment insurance and his family was only saved from the workhouse by a kind landlady who allowed the family to stay rent-free in their rooms. They must have been similar to the kind of families who Eleanor Rathbone was observing in Liverpool: families pushed into destitution not because of unwillingness to work but because of the unwillingness of the state to improve social conditions and services. Eventually, he obtained a job on the railways.

I never knew my paternal grandparents. I have many memories of my maternal ones, however. My grandmother had been in domestic service and told me stories of how she ironed the newspaper so that there were no creases in it when read by the master and mistress. She possessed a great fear of destitution and would plead, "Don't let me finish in the Union" (Union being the Poor Law Unions: that is, the workhouse). My grandfather was a horses man in more ways than one. He had driven horse-drawn buses and, in retirement enjoyed being an illegal bookie's runner.

I was born in 1936, in rented rooms in Ilford. My father endured some unemployment before borrowing the money to buy an old van which he then used to arrive early at London's vegetable markets where he bought fruit and vegetables for the local shops. He later used it for removals and made enough money to put down a deposit on a house – on a busy road, opposite a transport cafe, where he took his breaks. My father was hardworking, strict but with a great sense of humour. My mother was similarly hardworking: she not only loved and looked after the children and home, but also dealt with callers who wanted their furniture moved.

When war broke out in September 1939, I was among the hundreds of children who gathered at Ilford station with our gas masks and labels around our necks. I can only remember feeling ill in the very crowded train. My older sister looked after me and we went to Ipswich where billets were found for us. Our stay was no more than a few months. The bombs never came and we returned home. My father's lorry had been requisitioned and he had been drafted into a nearby war factory making parts for planes.

In September 1940, the bombs came with a vengeance. The docks and factories of East London were a prime target. For 76 consecutive nights, with one exception for very bad weather, the bombs descended, killing hundreds of people. One night, as we returned from our shelter in the garden, I looked at a London skyline which was completely red. It must have been 9 December when 1,600 fires raged.

After a long day at his factory bench, my father worked as an ARP (Air Raid Patrol) warden. During raids, wardens searched for incendiary bombs. After the all-clear, they joined other civil defence staff in digging out the dead and wounded. It was a harrowing task and my father found some compensation in the friendship of his colleagues. He would often invite the wardens into our home for a game of cards. I heard him telling them how he entered one bombed house where a woman promptly took down her underwear and asked him to pick the glass out of her backside. His friends roared with laughter. My mother was not so amused.

One night the nearby Co-op store was obliterated. Our windows and tiles were blasted. Reluctantly it was agreed that my father must stay while my mother would go away with my sister and myself. Our wider family was close knit, with grandparents, aunts and uncles who lived nearby and who constantly saw each other. Then there were relatives who lived outside and who we knew less well. We tried living with them in Leighton Buzzard, Brentwood and the village of Heronsgate – the latter having no internal running water. The homes proved too small for two families, so we returned home. More bombs came, and my parents turned back to the official evacuation scheme and we found ourselves in Cranleigh, Surrey. I did not know it, but it was very close to Lady Allen's residence in Hurtwood. Here, in the autumn of 1941, I started school. It consisted of a large, crowded, noisy hall. Each class sat around a table close by another class. I took a dislike to school, except for the break when we got free milk with a straw.

After a year, I never understood why, we moved on again. This time to a small hamlet called Cross Keys, a few miles outside of Hereford. We were billeted in a farm labourer's cottage with an outside, smelly toilet. As the nearest school was some miles away, my mother refused to send us, despite the threats from the truancy officer. I enjoyed roaming the fields with local children, scrumping and laughing with Italian prisoners-of-war, who worked in the fields. My mother was lonely and, in the evenings, went to the pub where we sat outside.

The only 'fly' in our evacuee 'ointment' was the householder, a burly, bullying man who ruled his wife with physical violence. Our mother was not the type to be browbeaten by anyone – perhaps this was why we moved around so much. One morning, the man accused me of stealing his tomatoes and wanted to 'belt' me. My mother retorted that it was not me, it was the rats and if anyone was going to hit her son it would be her. He sneered that rats gnawed tomatoes, not removed them. Good point. My mother promptly gathered us together and walked out: home again.

At home my new baby brother was born. Then came the flying bombs, the so-called doodlebugs, followed by the terrifying rockets. In November 1944, I came home from school to find that one had dropped close to our home. I scrambled into what was left of our house until I felt a hand on my shoulder, "It's alright, son". It was my father. My mother and the baby were in hospital. My sister and I moved in with our grandparents. When, eventually, my mother and my baby brother recovered, my father packed us off with instructions not to return until the war was over. We went to Hastings where we attended a school overcrowded with evacuees. For the first time I experienced others' anti-evacuee feelings. The 'vaccees' and the local children did not mix and the teachers seemed quick to punish the Londoners. Backward at the lessons, unhappy in a harsh school, our family living in one upstairs room with one bed, I was relieved when, in 1945, we went home for good.

I was just one of several million people who experienced the evacuation. It was a turning point for child care in Britain. The local authorities who received the children had to appoint child care visitors. A child care occupation was developed. Academics like Susan Issacs investigated what made for good foster homes (Issacs, 1941). Clare Winnicott highlighted the residential care of children in hostels. Dr Donald Winnicott became a regular broadcaster, advising foster parents how to cope with the children and natural parents how to deal with their loss. The government acknowledged that provision would have to be made for 'residual evacuees'; that is, children whose parents were dead or missing. The care of separated children was back on the national agenda. Then Lady Allen emerged as the leader of a campaign which, as I have explained, led to the famous 1948 Children Act that established local authority Children's Departments. A number of the first children's officers were women who had earned their child care spurs during the evacuation.

The evacuation must have left its mark on individual evacuees. Looking back, I can identify three elements which were significant for me. First, family unity became important. I was separated from my father for much of the war but I knew it was not of his choosing. I appreciated the courage of my mother who cared for us in difficult circumstances. Second, I never forgot the sense of isolation, even fear, in being a 'vaccee' outsider in Hastings. Third, knowing neighbours who were killed, I sometimes pondered what happened after death. My mother told me not to worry about such things. Yet I have always considered that this earthly life is not the full story. A belief in family unity, sympathy for those who felt alienated, a longing for some sort of spirituality. These themes have remained with me.

The route to child care (1946-61)

On returning to Ilford, I went to South Park junior school. I remember being embarrassed that I could neither say the alphabet nor tell the time. Indeed, I was so 'backward' that I was kept back a year and parted from my friends. At least I played in the school's cup-winning football side. In that extra and final year at junior school, like Peter Townsend, I benefited from a devoted teacher who gave me much individual attention. Even so, I failed the 11-plus examination, but passed at a second attempt. I thus proceeded to a new grammar school made possible by the war-time 1944 Education Act.

Soon after, a friend invited me to a Christian youth club called Covenanters. I went mainly because of its games night and sport. It gave me the first holidays of my childhood, and it also introduced me to Christianity, for I had never been sent to church. I gained much from the two leaders who talked with me and, for years after, offered me guidance and support. The junior schoolteacher and the club leaders had an important influence on me. They gave me a personal relationship outside of my immediate family. Interestingly, the need for such individual relationships was being made a cornerstone of the new Children's Departments under leaders like Barbara Kahan. Of course, this was quite unknown to me but years later I too tried to make personal relationships the foundation of community projects.

Initially I fared badly at grammar school. None of my street friends were there. But my liking for sport gained me acceptance. The system was for your class teacher to stay with you for the whole five years and I was fortunate enough to have one of the few who did not rely on the cane to keep order. My father wanted me to leave at the age of 16 and to get a safe job as a clerk. The teachers encouraged me to stay on and I gained good A levels and a state scholarship. I was not sure if I wanted to go to university. All my friends were at work and so I took a job in the Post Office Contracts Department until I was called up for national service in the RAF.

Like John Stroud, the RAF was a turning point for me; like John, I enjoyed the communal life. Like him, I was a fighter plotter/radar operator based on a coastal station. But I was the despair of the drill sergeant for I am tone deaf, and unable to pick out rhythm. "Holman", he bellowed, after another disastrous parade in which I could not keep in step, "You are a zombie. You can't help it but you are a zombie. Don't ever come on parade again". So, to the envy of my fellow airmen, during subsequent drills I was banished to sit on the beach. The RAF also introduced me to the British class system. I had never met anyone from private schools. Now I met officers – commonly known as "public school twits" – whose superior position stemmed from social background rather than ability. Simultaneously, I mixed with graduates who told me about university life. I decided to go.

I did not enjoy University College, London. History, economics and languages did not satisfy me. The cricket team nicknamed me 'Bertie' after an Australian cricketer, not because of my cricketing skill, but because they decided that my nasal London accent sounded Australian. I retreated into an insular Christianity, apart from the time I gave to helping at a youth club, and I must often have come across as withdrawn. I completed the degree and immediately transferred to the London School of Economics (LSE) for the certificate in social administration. Before I went, I undertook a placement in the Children's Department of Essex, located in an office at the back of a cinema in Romford. This was followed by a period working in a children's home. I had found what I wanted to do. Then, while browsing in the local library, I came across a collection of essays. I was gripped by one written by a Peter Townsend (Townsend, 1958). He presented an analysis of poverty along with solutions to be found in action by the Labour Party. Even more, I was moved by his insistence that socialism was more than politics and was a set of beliefs which had to be applied to the way we lived as individuals. Peter Townsend reissued the essay in 1973 and I wish it could be republished today with its clarion call, "You cannot live like a lord and preach as a socialist" (Townsend, 1973, p 21).

The certificate course from 1960-61 was a revelation. Professor Richard Titmuss and his young team, which included Peter Townsend, Brian Abel-Smith and David Donnison, were passionate about social conditions, inequality and the social services. Until then, my sympathies for the alienated and my dislike of the establishment had lacked a political focus. Now I became a socialist. During the course, my tutor advised me to undertake the professional training in social work so I applied, and was accepted, for the diploma in applied social studies.

During the summer vacation, I was sent to work in a training home for mothers. It was run by a stern superintendent – "doors locked at 9 pm" – and his wife, the matron, who taught cookery, budgeting and child care to the so-called 'problem mothers'. Within a few days, the superintendent had a breakdown and walked out with his wife. I promptly telephoned County Hall where a senior officer calmly told me to hang on for a few days while she organised replacements. Young and green, I certainly could not teach cooking and baby care and I definitely could not appease the women, some of whom began to bring in their boyfriends. However, some of the women took pity on me. They provided me with meals, they kicked out the boyfriends and they organised the place. I received my first lessons about the abilities of people who are too often cast by the social services into the roles of inadequate clients.

Once on the 'generic course', as the applied social studies diploma was called, I found many of the casework classes – which involved examining case interactions between social workers and clients in enormous Freudian detail – to be incredibly boring. Some of the lectures were so dry that I stopped going and went off to play hockey, my latest sport. The course was enlivened by the teaching of Clare Winnicott, who conveyed a passion for child care. Her lectures were carefully prepared and well-delivered. By contrast, Donald Winnicott shuffled into the room without any notes and drew 'a squiggle' on the blackboard. After asking students what they could see in it, he produced lessons from children he had been seeing in his practice. He was not as easy to follow as Clare but he clearly shared her concern for deprived children and her conviction that child care officers could be of help to them.

The 'generic course' required students to pass two closely supervised casework placements. My first was in a probation office in North London. I went with an attractive Scottish student, Annette Leishman, and soon we were 'going steady'. My second placement was in Chelmsford with the Essex Children's Department, where I was supervised by Ursula Behr, a founding member of the Association of Child Care Officers (ACCO) and a gentle, concerned and astute supervisor. At the the end of my time there, Annette and I took Ursula to see Lionel Bart's musical, *Blitz*. Ursula wept. We did not know that she had been a pre-war refugee from Germany.

Inspired by Clare Winnicott's mission, I wanted nothing more than to join a Children's Department. Clare Winnicott did not regard child care as a job, but as a vocation. She had the same sense of mission that informed the energy of Barbara Kahan and the persistence of John Stroud. I was accepted by the Children's Department of Hertfordshire County Council and Annette – we got engaged sitting in Russell Square the day our examinations finished – went to work at Barnet General Hospital as a medical social worker.

Children's Departments (1962-66)

At Hertfordshire, I was sent to the office in Welwyn Garden City where the area officer, Vera Roberts, gave me an office no bigger than a cupboard and a caseload of over 100. She also announced that, as I was so inexperienced, she had arranged for me to have 'digs' with a foster family.

The foster home was marvelous. The foster mother was young and lively. The foster father, too, was affectionate with the children, but he thought me an idiot to take such a low-paid job while an unqualified person like himself was earning three times as much as a salesman. The first night I was given a bedroom with a young boy. He asked me whether I wanted the top or bottom bunk. We had had bunks at home so, being aware of the likelihood of tumbling out of the top one, I opted for the bottom bunk. During the night, I was awoken by a steady drip, drip, drip on my face. In the morning, the foster mother laughingly said, "That's your first lesson in child care. Never sleep beneath an enuretic child".

I was soon to learn another lesson. Their second foster child, a 10-year-old girl, eagerly anticipated visits from her natural mother and wept if she failed to appear. Sometimes her mother came with 'an uncle'. The foster mother was critical of the natural mother's morals and argued that, as the visits (or lack of them) upset the girl, they should be stopped altogether. I began to agree. Then I found other accommodation and concentrated on my own caseload. I was alone in the office one evening when the distressed foster mother telephoned to say that the girl had run away. I searched the city for her and finally found her in the library. She ran into my arms and sobbed, "I want my mum".

The incident taught me the importance to children of their natural parents even when the latter upset societal norms. The lesson was reinforced by my supervisor, John Stroud. He told me to read one of the few studies on the subject, namely *The self image of the foster child* by the American, Eugene Weinstein, who showed that foster children fared better when they had full understanding of their own backgrounds, and when they were in regular contact with their natural parents (Weinstein, 1960). My child care practice changed. I began to initiate discussions about natural parents with children in care, their foster parents and residential

carers. With John Stroud's encouragement, I undertook a small study of
my own on the relationship between foster children and their parents.
But my life was not confined to work. I joined, and was soon an office
holder, in the local Labour Party. But child care could not be separated
from politics. As a member of ACCO, I joined its campaign in support of
the eventual 1963 Children and Young Persons Act which gave statutory
backing to local authorities to prevent children being needlessly removed
from their parents and placed in public care. The years that followed
witnessed child care staff developing strategies to implement the Act and
I recall hearing the dynamic Barbara Kahan lecturing on this subject.
Simultaneously, as a political activist, I could join in the pressure on the
government to supply the resources for these strategies. In addition, I
became involved in leading a church youth club, with Annette active with
the girl members. On one occasion we chartered a plane, an old Dakota,
literally tied together with string, to take 40 to a camp in Jersey. We were
accompanied by Laurie Laken, another former evacuee, with whom I
have been friends since boyhood. He went to work in approved schools
and later in community youth work. At the camp he displayed his great
skill of being able to maintain friendships with young people while still
keeping order. The youth clubs too were not entirely separate from my
work for they involved some young people who were in care.

Most importantly, Annette and I were married, and Ruth was born in
1965, David in 1966. Yet even family life was not completely split off from
work. We were living in a terraced corporation house located in the
midst of my 'patch'. I had placed a child for adoption with a couple in
the next street. Children on my caseload would sometimes drop in – I am
still in touch with one nearly four decades later. Without meaning to do
so, I was experiencing child care in the community, which was to become
a major part of our lives in later years.

A job in child care, a young family, running a youth club, a political
activist – life was demanding and stimulating. Then, by accident, my job
changed. One day, I received a letter which contained details about a
lectureship for a university child care course. I was certainly interested in
research and had delivered a few talks to local groups on child care, but I
considered myself too inexperienced to think about lecturing. I threw
the details into the waste paper basket. Later, when I emptied the contents
of the basket into the dustbin, I spotted a hand-written letter clipped to
the back of the circular. It was from Professor Richard Titmuss suggesting
that I apply for the post. I had never realised that Richard Titmuss had
even noticed me. I discussed the job with the children's officer, Sylvia

Watson, who explained that Hertfordshire was to start an emergency child care course at Stevenage College of Further Education, not far from our home, and that I should apply for the post of assistant tutor.

My time at Stevenage was short but very worthwhile. The child care course was located in one room in a pre-fab hut. Staff were not expected to do research – which was a disappointment for me – and there was no office. But there was an appealing kind of social mixing. Unlike at most universities, staff and students shared the same dining room and played in the same cricket team. Tutors taught evening courses to the general public. The emergency two-year child care course was for 'mature' students with no formal qualifications. They were deeply committed to their change of career and I formed long-term friendships with some of them. Bron, for example, was an outspoken former nurse who introduced herself with, "Hello, I'm Bron Soan. I'm a socialist and atheist". She used to laugh at my Christianity but our mutual socialism drew us together. She proved a first-rate social worker and years later became a Christian. She then divided her time between social work in Britain and working in El Salvador in difficult and dangerous circumstances. As a pensioner, she has taken kids from Easterhouse, where I now live, for holidays.

John Stroud had applied to be the tutor in charge of the Stevenage course and both he and I were disappointed when he did not get it. He was not resentful, however, and the appointed course leader, Colin Akhurst, and I helped John with *ACCORD* and eventually took over as joint editors. I also renewed contact with Clare Winnicott who was in charge of the emergency courses. The course tutors used to gather periodically to meet with her in London where she made child care training sound like the world's most important venture.

The 1960s were probably the high point of the Children's Departments. Certainly, they had many limitations. In particular, some local authorities were so small that their tiny Children's Departments could not provide a range of services and were considered to be of lower status than the larger Education and Health Departments. Despite the appointment of some exceptional residential staff, children's homes were largely run by unqualified personnel. Sadly, much child abuse probably went unrecognised. In many ways, however, the departments were a new and effective force for child care. In a previous chapter, attention was given to what Barbara Kahan saw as the achievements of the Children's Departments. I agree with her and wish to add three more:

- The Children's Departments promoted a form of care which can only be described as personal. The Curtis Report had declared that it placed "great importance to establishing and maintaining a continuing personal relationship between the child deprived of a home and the official of the local authority responsible for ... him"(Home Office, Ministry of Health and Ministry of Education, 1946, para 445). Many elected members and appointed officials took this to heart. Local councillors often gave much time to visiting children's homes, where they got to know children as individuals. Children's officers, including those in charge of large departments, sometimes carried caseloads themselves so that they did not lose touch with children. Above all, child care officers saw their responsibility and their skill as knowing, caring for and communicating with children. This personal approach was developed within the sphere of local government which, up to then, had often been identified with the impersonal approach of form filling, regulation and bureaucracy.
- The Children's Departments brought natural parents into the state child care process. In the past, deprived children had often been 'rescued' from their parents, with both the Poor Law agencies and voluntary societies acting on the belief that, if the parents ceded the care of their children, then they were failures who should have no more influence over them. This view was challenged by people like Barbara Kahan, John Stroud and Clare Winnicott, who demonstrated, first, that separated children usually benefited from contact with their natural families and that, second, the parents often did love them and wanted them back.
- Importantly, the Children's Departments developed field workers who were specialists in child care. Previously, local authority responsibility for deprived children had been fragmented between a number of services whose main duties were for education, health and destitution. The Children's Departments could concentrate on separated children while the government established child care courses which were led by specialists like Clare Winnicott. The outcome was that many child care officers were skilled in such matters as reception into care, fostering, adoption, family casework and prevention. They became adept at negotiating on behalf of children and their families with agencies which included Housing Departments, Education Departments, the courts, the police and the National Assistance Board. In particular, they were skilled at understanding and relating to the children. Despite long hours, large caseloads and very modest salaries, they retained a sense of enthusiasm and commitment. As one officer – who had previously

spent years in the police force – put it, "There was a sense of mission. I could not have left child care and gone to something else" (Holman, 1998, p 98).

Research

While a new child care officer, I visited a foster mother who told me that aliens were sending radio waves to kill her. When I asked the area officer what we could do about her foster child, she replied briskly, "Nothing, CLP". I thought this was something to do with the Communist Party until she explained that CLP (Child Life Protection) was the Victorian language still applied to private foster care. On my caseload I had several private fosterings which occurred when parents (not public agencies) selected foster parents for their children. Although the placements were not made by the Children's Departments, they did have a duty to visit the foster children from time to time.

Almost nothing was written about private fostering and its 10,000 notified private foster children. The subject became my PhD and took years to complete. I researched and wrote it when my two children were small, while lecturing and while still giving some time to youth work. Annette said it was our 'third child' and certainly I could not have completed it without her practical support. The study established that private foster children were of three main kinds, those placed by West Africans who had come to Britain to study and placed their children in foster homes so that they could earn money in the evenings, by single parents and by deserted spouses. Although some capable private foster parents were identified, the research detected a number of very unsuitable ones – including some with their own children in public care. On a number of emotional, educational and physical measures, the private foster children tended to fare worse than matched children from a sample of children in the care of Children's Departments. Links between the private foster children and their natural parents were often tenuous. Sometimes the children were hundreds of miles from their parents and grew up hardly knowing them. Child care officers visited private foster children far less frequently than those in public care, despite the fact that they were often in conditions which placed them at risk of neglect. They considered that their duties towards the private foster parents were too vague and that their powers to intervene were too limited.

Trading in children: A study of private fostering was published in 1973

(Holman, 1973). It gained some coverage in the press and one popular Sunday newspaper offered me a large sum for my files so that it could expose the foster parents. Needless to say, I declined. Questions were asked in Parliament and the government promised to look into the matter but nothing happened. I had proposed that local authorities should have greater powers and resources both to control and support the private foster parents, that the children should be visited as regularly as children in public care, and that the authorities should have a duty to visit the natural parents in order to encourage continued contacts. A few minor reforms did follow but, if anything, the situation today has deteriorated. The government has even ceased its practice of issuing figures about the numbers of private foster children. In 1997, an official review by Sir William Utting of the safeguards for children living away from home was issued. He concluded that "Private fostering is clearly an area where children are not being safeguarded properly, indeed an unknown number are likely to be seriously at risk" (DoH, 1997, p 44). A year later, the government took further action to safeguard many groups of vulnerable children, but declined to act on Utting's proposal for a register of private foster children (DoH, 1998b, p 20).

The private fostering study also allowed me to continue my interest in the involvement of natural parents in fosterings. The study concerned the sizeable number of 246 private foster and local authority foster children. I was able to examine the way in which the foster parents regarded fostering, in particular whether they saw themselves as replacing the natural parents or working with them. In addition, I looked at the effects on the children of the amount of, and the nature of, their contact with their natural parents. From this I was able to conceptualise two kinds of fostering: exclusive fostering in which the foster parents wanted to contain the foster child within their family while keeping out the child's relatives and statutory agencies; and inclusive fosterings in which the foster parents offered care while being ready to draw in other parties of the fostering complex. I pointed to the tension between the fact that most local authority foster parents seemed to favour the exclusive concept, although research studies indicated that the inclusive concept was associated with many favourable outcomes for the children (Holman, 1975).

Face to face with poverty

In 1967, I went to the University of Birmingham as a lecturer in social work. The course was a generic social work one, in which I taught most of the child care component. These were the years in which the organisational reform of the social services was the big social work issue. In Scotland, the 1968 Social Work (Scotland) Act established local authority social work departments. The Seebohm Report, covering England and Wales, was published in 1968 and many social workers joined the Seebohm Implementation Group to persuade the government to amalgamate varied specialist services into one local authority social services department – which happened in 1970. I did not join and I was present when Clare Winnicott spoke at the final meeting of ACCO. I shared some of her fears that the abolition of the Children's Departments might lead to the loss of the strengths of specialist child care officers. However, I was enthusiastic about the chapters on community and prevention in the Seebohm Report (Home Office, Ministry of Education and Science, Ministry of Housing and Local Government and Ministry of Health, 1968, chs 14 and 16). My social horizons were broadening, although, I fear, I was not sufficiently sensitive towards colleagues who did not share them. I changed from being a lecturer in social work to one in social administration.

It was in Birmingham that our children, Ruth and David, started school. And it was in Birmingham that I came face to face with poverty. I joined a committee which was setting up an adventure playground in the multi-racial, very deprived area of Handsworth. I took advice from Marjory Allen over the telephone. The playground was successfully launched under the leadership of Dee Newton. Later, I participated in the founding of the Handsworth Day Care Centre. I also played for the local football team, Soho United, which was made up mainly of people of Irish extraction and Afro-Caribbeans. But I was an outsider. I travelled in from a more comfortable suburb and I recall a member of the militant Black Panthers telling me that I was "a white missionary". Nonetheless, I was able to see at first hand the deprivations and injustices imposed on black people. These were the years of Enoch Powell's 'Rivers of Blood' speech. I played a small part in attacking this racism and received hate mail from racists. Even more disturbing was my discovery of racial prejudice within the church. The church we attended was socially active, had youth organisations which our children enjoyed, and saw itself as upholding biblical Christianity. Certainly, we met some gracious people there. It was located in a road which contained a large number of black people. Yet few stayed in the church. I spoke on this issue at a meeting there and I recall an elderly man jumping to his feet, declaring that he had been all over the world, that Britain was the best country and we should keep it as it was. He was loudly applauded. I felt alienated from the church. I should add that the church contained one young man who coped with this better than me. Andrew Funnell had been brought up in the church and he and his future wife Margaret became our long-standing friends. He entered the ministry and they have always made a stand against racism and have now served in the same Merseyside area for over a quarter of a century.

We became friendly with a number of Handsworth families and soon became aware of their extreme poverty. Of course, in my childhood and as a child care officer I had met a number of families with very low incomes. I was familiar with the studies by Peter Townsend but I had never come across such dreadful living conditions. One, woman, Maureen, and her husband and three children lived in two rooms in a privately rented basement. A third room was unusable because of the damp. They shared an outside toilet with other tenants. The sole means of heating was by leaving open the door of the cooker. The husband's low wages meant that they could not afford a mortgage or a higher rent. They were low down on the council's housing list. In despair, Maureen tried to gas herself but was saved by the arrival of a friend. She collected her kids and arrived on our doorstep. She stayed until a housing association was persuaded to take them in.

Experiences like these taught me that poverty was far worse than I had previously appreciated. They also reinforced my understanding that poor people were not inadequate. Maureen had been a helper in a local playgroup until poverty forced her almost to take her own life. Next I began to see the connection between poverty and family malfunctioning. Annette obtained a research post with the remarkable Harriett Wilson, who had played a prominent part in setting up the Child Poverty Action Group (CPAG). With an educational psychologist, Geoffrey Herbert, Harriett initiated an extensive study of how poverty affects child and parent behaviour in large families. The study was unusual in that it had a control group of families who were not poor. Annette was the interviewer who periodically visited and interviewed the families. The results showed that many of the poor parents did not use the child-rearing methods associated with developing the social and educational skills of their children who, therefore, grew to be at a disadvantage. However, the parents' deficiencies did not spring from a lack of love, nor from ignorance about good parenting, nor from not holding the same values as more affluent families. Rather, their poverty restricted the kind of parenting they wanted to give. The poorer parents could not participate in play, outings and holidays because they lacked money. They could not afford the books and toys which stimulated intellectual growth. In overcrowded homes with thin walls and no gardens, the children inevitably spent much time on the streets. Not least, tensions over money and bad health added to the pressures on parenting. When *Parents and children in the inner city* appeared, it confirmed in research form the observation of Eleanor Rathbone, some 60 years earlier, that such families needed not lessons in 'mother craft', but decent incomes and conditions (Wilson and Herbert, 1978).

These experiences had three important effects on me. First, I introduced welfare rights teaching onto the social work courses with which I was involved. Further, I advocated that social workers should back and cooperate with local community projects which were supplying day care, youth clubs, holidays and other practical services which residents wanted.

Second, I advocated that much more attention should be given to what poor people were saying. Far from being inadequate, social services' users often know more about the situation than the officials. I encouraged Maureen to write and she had a moving and profound article published in *New Society* (Maureen, 1971). I attended a conference addressed by Sir Keith Joseph, the Conservative Secretary of State for Social Services. Sir Keith was voicing his cycle of deprivation theory in which he saw inadequate parents spawning the next generation of inadequate families. I challenged him to listen to what these parents were actually saying and, to his credit, he promptly invited me to bring some parents to meet him. The meeting took place in his London offices and he listened carefully as they explained that it was difficult to be poor and to live up to the parental standards he was setting. Sir Keith then came to visit the Handsworth Day Care Centre. Again, he was charming and interested. He was impressed by the fact that local residents were committee members. Yet he made strange statements. He asked me to walk with him through the streets of Handsworth and probed me about the number of Irish immigrants. In all seriousness, he asked what could be done to stop them breeding like rabbits. He seemed to have a fear that, because poor people had more children than the affluent, eventually their stock would over-run that of their 'betters'.

Third, the content of my writings began to shift. I still wrote about child care but, in addition, I studied poverty in more depth and began to grasp more fully that the explanation of poverty rested not in individual laziness, not in cycles of deprivation and not in the deficiencies of welfare agencies. Between 1972-74, I was senior lecturer in social administration at the University of Glasgow. For the first time in my adult life, I was not involved in running youth clubs, although I still helped at one. I spent more time with our children as we explored Glasgow, which is Annette's hometown. It also gave me more time to understand just what was behind poverty. As I expressed in *Poverty: Explanations of social deprivation*, poverty stems from the unequal structures of society which means that the resources of power, income and wealth are constantly denied to one section of the population (Holman, 1978). I believe that the removal of poverty requires radical political action. But this does not mean that poverty was irrelevant to child care. It became clear to me that poverty was closely associated with the numbers of children who entered public care. In a pamphlet, written for CPAG, I brought together the evidence to demonstrate the link between poverty and reception into care. It followed that the prevention of children's removal from their families required not just skilled social work, but also social policies which countered poverty (Holman, 1976). Child care and poverty reform went together.

Promoting prevention (1974-76)

In 1974, I was invited to apply for the new chair of social policy at the University of Bath. Annette obtained a post as lecturer in social work at the University of Bristol. We moved into our first detached house in a safe cul-de-sac while the children settled happily into the new junior school.

As I will explain, I did not fit in as a university professor. However, I found that the position gave me a voice on matters of social policy and I focused on the child care issues of prevention and permanency. In my early years as a child care officer, John Stroud had taught me the importance of children retaining links with their natural parents. He perceived that preventing children having to leave their families was the best way of maintaining such links. Barbara Kahan had campaigned for local authorities to have the legal powers to undertake prevention. Thereafter, I was one of many child care officers who attempted to put prevention into practice.

Following the creation of social services departments (SSDs) and social work departments (SWDs), fears were expressed that preventative activity by social workers had declined. Professor Roy Parker chaired a working party, of which I was a member, which stated, "At present prevention is a tree of stunted growth" (Parker, 1980, p 59). Some former child care enthusiasts thought that prevention had withered because child care skills were less in evidence. But there were other explanations. A major one was that social services began to give priority to finding permanent substitute families for children in care. In 1973, Maria Colwell suffered an horrific death at the hands of her stepfather. She had been in the care of the East Sussex SSD which had not opposed her mother's application to a court for a revocation of the care order. The mass media furiously accused social workers of worshipping 'the blood tie' and keeping children with unsuitable parents. Parents of children in care became objects of condemnation. The implication was that social workers should give more attention to removal and less to prevention.

In 1973, two respected social work figures, Jane Rowe and Lydia Lambert, published *Children who wait*, in which they estimated that 6,000 children in care were being allowed to drift without decisions being made for their permanent futures (Rowe and Lambert, 1973). The study became ammunition for a growing pro-adoption lobby. In a study of the book and its influence, Greg Kelly explains that its figures actually suggest that the social workers – from whom information was obtained about the children – considered that far more children needed permanent or indefinite foster homes than adoption (Kelly, 1998, pp 54, 59). Nonetheless, at a time when there was a growing shortage of babies for adoption and when social workers were being urged to remove more children, the book stimulated the permanency movement.

Also published in 1973 was an American book by Joseph Goldstein, Anna Freud and Albert Solnit, which drew on psychoanalytic theory to assert that children could not relate satisfactorily to two sets of parent figures: natural and substitute. They continued that, once in care, children who could not be speedily returned to their own parents should be placed permanently with adopters (Goldstein et al, 1973, ch 3). These writers gave theoretical justification to the drive to remove and permanently place children away from their parents. As Kelly stated, "The permanence movement dominated thinking about children in long-term care for 15 years.... Almost all local authorities and voluntary agencies developed permanence policies" (Kelly, 1998, pp 56, 59). The 1975 Children Act gave local authorities greater powers to remove children from their parents and extended the grounds on which their consent to adoption could be dispensed.

Not all child care social workers agreed with this trend. Indeed, social work was divided into two camps, one emphasising prevention, the other, permanence. Lorraine Fox Harding, in a later book, applies the titles of "the kinship defenders" and "the society as parent protagonists" and goes into detail about the arguments of both (Fox Harding, 1991). I supported the former view. In a fruitless lobby to modify the draconian 1975 Children Bill, I met Jane Streather of CPAG, Jo Tunnard who became director of the Family Rights Group, and Jane Tunstill, later to be a professor of child care studies. The arguments we put forward included the following:

• Children were best cared for by their own parents and families. Even when removed, most still benefited from regular contact with and, at least, full knowledge about their relatives.
• Prevention had not been fully implemented. It followed that some children were being permanently placed away from natural parents who might well have coped given more effective social work support.
• Most children taken into care were those of poor parents. The 1975 Children Bill contained no provisions for parents who could have kept their children if given higher incomes.

These arguments were not original. They were repeating many of the points made by Eleanor Rathbone, Barbara Kahan, John Stroud and Peter Townsend. The difference was that they were being presented in different circumstances, at a time when the media focus on child abuse and uncaring and feckless parents was pushing local authorities and central government to develop policies and practices which made it even harder for socially deprived families to survive.

The differences between the two sides must not be overstated. Certainly, Jane Rowe is an advocate and indeed an expert on fostering as well as adoption. The support for the hard line taken by Goldstein, Freud and Solnit melted somewhat as a succeeding book made overt their right-wing political position of opposition to state welfare expenditure on the grounds that it weakened families' sense of responsibility. They saw adoption as cheaper than other forms of care (Goldstein et al, 1979). Those in the prevention school were not opposed to adoption. I have placed a number of children with prospective adoptees. I know from experience with many troubled children that not all adoptions work out successfully. But many do provide happy upbringings. My wish is not to undermine adoptions, but rather to ensure that all parents, especially lone parents, receive the material, social and emotional support to help them in bringing up their children. In short, if they do decide to place their children for adoption it should not be because social deprivations force them into that position.

Since the passing of the 1975 Children Act, the practice of prevention has waxed and waned. For a time, statutory social work was marked by an authoritarian, interventionist style towards parents suspected of child abuse. As David Thorpe has shown, as more child abuse inquiries followed, so SSDs shifted ever more resources towards child protection and away from prevention (Thorpe, 1994). But prevention never disappeared. A number of voluntary child care societies developed family centres as a means of supporting vulnerable families. The 1989 Children Act in England and Wales and the 1995 Children Act (Scotland) in Scotland seek to ensure that children are given protection while local authorities have the green light to support families. Of course, this is not to say that the SSDs and SWDs have the resources for these ends. Nor does it mean that the poverty which grinds down so many parents has been removed. The more balanced approach, as expressed in the 1989 Act, is well represented in the work of the British Agencies for Adoption and Fostering which, under its capable director Felicity Collier, strives to promote high standards in adoption and fostering. In 2001, the Labour government is proposing a new adoption Act which will increase and speed up the number of adoptions and improve adoption services. In cases where adoption is not appropriate for the children involved, it is likely that a new special guardianship order will give greater security to the children's carers while not legally cutting the children's ties with their parents. Few social workers will disagree with these provisions, but the proposal that permanency planning will begin six months *after* children enter care and the absence of any proposals to increase resources for prevention – or family support, as it is now called – show that the permanency movement is again in the ascendancy. Meanwhile, the Conservatives wish to go further; as their former leader, William Hague stated, "We will introduce much tougher requirements on local authorities to put children up for adoption.... Ideally, we would like every child to at least be considered for adoption" (Hague, 1999).

In 1976, I resigned from my university chair. The reasons were complex. I was not an efficient manager and found the numerous university committee meetings and the piles of paperwork to be unfulfilling. Simultaneously, I felt some guilt that I was separated from the practice of social work. I was teaching social work students and writing books, but I was not practising what I preached. In addition, I was anxious to develop prevention. It was not just that I was disappointed that prevention seemed to be held in less regard by social workers. It was also that I was realising that preventing family break-ups, avoiding children having to go into care and diverting young people from delinquency might best be done from within deprived areas rather by outsiders who commuted in. Probably most important, however, was the resolution of my religious struggles.

In Birmingham, I had been progressively alienated from churches which I saw as upholders of the status quo. But my criticisms and drifting away did not make me a better Christian. On the contrary, I became increasingly self-centred, wanted more money and wanted to be seen as the 'young professor'. In fact, I became like the very people I had criticised: which was hypocritical. I achieved academic status, got the detached house in a nice area, obtained an affluent lifestyle. But it did not satisfy me. In my last years in Birmingham, I studied the Bible. I studied the 'minor prophets' and believe that Christianity is about loving God and loving our neighbours. In Bath, I became fascinated by the lifestyle of Jesus Christ, who is said to have lived modestly, shared his goods with the poor, and attacked the establishment. After talks with my wife – always a better Christian than me – I left university in order to initiate a community project.

The Southdown Project (1976-86)

In 1976, we moved a couple of miles to a house alongside the Southdown Council Estate; our children did not even have to change their junior schools. I had obtained a small amount of funding from a charitable trust for a community child care project and the Church of England Children's Society (as it was then called) agreed to administer it. The aims were to provide youth amenities, to prevent children being taken into care, and to help potential and actual delinquents. It had one worker, myself, a small budget, and its basis was simply that I should live there.

I was determined to listen to what residents wanted and I started by knocking on every door on the estate. One woman leant out of a window and shouted, "If you're the bleeding welfare, clear off". Fortunately, most people welcomed the chance to give their opinions, with most asking me to provide something for local children who roamed the streets. In the evenings, I hung about, often feeling nervous and threatened, and listened to teenagers as they moaned about being bored.

I got to know Dave Wiles who had lived in Southdown all his life. His father had spent many years in prison and Dave was unemployed and on probation for violence and drug offences. He was anxious, however, to put something back into an area where he had been feared. Dave became the first chair of a senior youth club and, within a year, I managed to raise the money for him to join the project. The youth club met in an old pre-fab, various church halls and our house. An old lean-to against the side of the house became the teenagers' own den where they could gather, mostly unsupervised, to chat, smoke and listen to music. The activities multiplied with junior youth clubs, outings, holidays, and individual counselling for young people and parents. Jane Sellars was appointed as another project worker and built up activities for girls and young women, while later another young man from the estate, Jim Davis, completed the team. In 1981, I published an account of the first three years (Holman, 1981). It showed that in those years there had been 1,596 knocks on the door, hence the title *Kids at the door.* Clearly, our home was under tremendous pressure.

Annette and our children – who were by then at secondary school – certainly had their lives disrupted as our home became part of the project. Annette had a full-time job, but she was often the one who let the teenagers into the lean-to in the evening. She joined with Jane Sellars in setting up a group for very young mothers who met in one room in the house while their babies were looked after in another room. However, there were some upsetting experiences. On one occasion we took in a woman and her children who had been physically assaulted by her husband. He banged loudly on our door and shouted that he had a right to see his children. I am a wimp but I pointed out that he had no right to hit them and refused him entrance. He drew back his fist and smashed it against the wall until his knuckles were bleeding. He stormed off cursing and threatening. As I closed the door, I saw our Ruth standing there white-faced. She was in the midst of her O level examinations.

Ruth and David went to the local comprehensives, joined in many activities and came to the annual camp at Norfolk. During one camp, I was contacted by a mother who gave me the tragic news that her husband had died suddenly of a heart attack. She asked me to say nothing to her son, to give him a good holiday and, on his return, to help her break the news to him. On the Saturday, I drove the minibus back to Southdown, dropped the other campers off and then stopped at our house to unload the sleeping bags. It had been burgled and ransacked. I then took the boy home where we broke the news of the death of his father as gently as we could. He just screamed. I returned to our home to await Annette, Ruth and David. They were all devastated that their rooms had been vandalised and their belongings taken. I discovered that it had been done by some teenagers from an adjoining estate who knew we would be away. I thought, "What am I doing to my family? Do I want to carry on?"

But we did carry on. A major reason was the support we received from neighbours. One man arrived with a television to replace the one that had been stolen. He had a criminal past himself but snorted that he would never steal from people like us. Young people came down and promised to beat up the villains – an offer which we declined. One of our dearest friends was a widow on a low income, who made her living as a church cleaner. She was a stalwart member of the Labour Party, always ready to do the foot slogging tasks, and a loyal supporter of the church. She, too, called, bringing cakes. I had come to help this community but, as the years went by, I was increasingly being helped by its members. Our family bonds, too, were close. The children did sometimes get fed up with answering the door or finding the home full of other children. Annette did sigh at the stains on the carpet and the broken furniture. But Annette and I always made time to be alone with our children. Today, as adults, Ruth and David feel that through these experiences they saw a side of life they would otherwise have missed and they now support those who are socially deprived. And our family links remain close.

After a few years, the house was bursting at its seams. Residents decided that the Southdown Project needed its own building. They raised half the money by fundraising events and applying to local charities, with The Children's Society (as it was by then called) giving the other half. It was built on a grassy slope next to the public toilets and opened in 1983. Dave Wiles had been seconded to take a diploma in social work at the University of Bristol and, on his return, he took over as leader, with myself as the assistant.

We continued for 10 years in Southdown. Years later, in 1998-99, I undertook a follow-up of 51 young people – by then in their thirties – with whom we had had the closest contacts and published the findings in *Kids at the door revisited* (Holman, 2000). Who were the 51 young people? When they first came to the project, nearly all were from low-income families; 57% experienced school difficulties such as suspensions and truancy; 39% were in trouble with the police; and 22% were in families visited by social workers. All these factors are associated with future educational failure, unemployment, crime and unstable relationships. Overall, 39% were at high risk, 22% at moderate risk and 29% at low risk according to an 'at risk' scale I devised for the study. Despite this, as teenagers, only one of them went into public care and, though some did have court appearances, none went into juvenile custody. I think the project did justify the claims, made years before by Barbara Kahan, that intensive involvement between staff and at-risk young people could avoid them having to enter public care, could divert them away from delinquency.

Just as important was to discover how they turned out as adults. Forty-seven per cent failed to obtain any educational qualifications and 18% endured periods of unemployment. By 1999, however, most of those available for work were in jobs, though usually low-paid or moderately paid jobs. Nearly all were in stable relationships. Fourteen per cent had been in serious trouble with the police although, it must be added, this had mostly occurred in early adulthood and none had experienced recent prison sentences. Eight per cent had been serious drinkers and 6% had problems of serious debt. On a satisfactory/unsatisfactory life scale, explained in the book, 14% were rated as unsatisfactory and 86% as satisfactory.

The outcomes were far better than could have been expected from the young people's early 'at-risk' factors. What made the difference? Obviously, many factors contributed including the availability of jobs, the support of their partners and, not least, their own personalities. Nonetheless, all the former young people were enthusiastic about the project and most indicated that it had played a significant part in their lives. One man had been frequently in trouble as a teenager. Now the manager of several shops, he looked back and said:

> Without the project I would almost certainly have got into more trouble. If I had been kicked out of school permanently what would have happened? What would have happened if I had been sent away? (Holman, 2000, p 68).

What was it about the Southdown Project that made its impact so great? According to those involved in it, the following five factors were crucial:

- The project provided clubs which diverted some bored youngsters away from trouble. In addition, our house was open to them as a place where they could always go for company, for shelter, for a chat. The lean-to became the teenagers' own club where they could meet apart from adults.
- The project offered help with individual relationships. Sixty-five per cent of the young people turned to the project leaders for help on matters such as delinquency, tensions with their parents, trouble at school,

difficulties at work, problems with boy/girlfriends. The relationships between the leaders and the youngsters were friendly but differed from everyday friendships, which are usually between two people in the same age group. I termed them 'resourceful friendships', in which emotions were felt and pleasure was gained from each other's company, but all within the context of an agency in which the relationships were made in order to achieve certain objectives – like reducing truancy – and which were based on certain principles, such as confidentiality (Holman, 2000, p 78).

- The project adopted a community approach. The project was open to any youngsters on the estate, not just to those with problems of crime, drug abuse and so on. It ran open youth clubs, sports teams and holidays. Consequently, it was never stigmatised as being just for 'problem kids'. Moreover, those teenagers who did have severe personal difficulties mixed with and were influenced by those who did not. The project also involved adults. Regular outings drew in families, while Bank holidays often brought games on the field in which young people took on parents. Many residents were then drawn in as volunteers and sessional workers and eventually became the committee which took over the project.

- The project staff lived in the area. The fact that we used the same shops, buses, churches and schools made us known to and gradually accepted by residents. We were able to acquire knowledge of local needs, weaknesses and strengths. Being on the spot, we were always available to adults and children in emergencies.

- The project was long-term. The staff were committed to staying for at least 10 years. We grew up with local families and were close to children as they grew into teenagers and then young adults. It was easier to relate to, and even control, some wild teenagers when we had known them as kids. Further, both teenagers and their parents revealed a growing trust as the years went by and were therefore more ready to turn to and confide in the project staff when in need.

I had kept in touch with a number of the young people for over 20 years. For others, going back meant that I was seeing them for the first time after a long absence. It was a moving experience, which culminated in a Southdown reunion party in the project building. One of the most gratifying findings was that 41% of the former young people had themselves participated in some form of youth work, usually as volunteers but in some instances as full-time workers. It seemed as though they had been helped by their involvement in the project and wanted to make a similar contribution as they grew older.

By 1986, I felt nicely redundant. The project was in the hands of local leadership, local volunteers and local committee members. Ruth and David were at college and, at the age of 50, I reckoned I had one more shot left in me. We decided to move back to Glasgow.

Easterhouse, child care and inequality (1987 onwards)

Annette obtained a post in the Pre-Fives Unit of Strathclyde Education Department and I obtained some part-time financial support from the National Children's Home. We moved into a second-floor flat in Easterhouse. At that time, Easterhouse was a largely council house estate with a population of 40,000. Since then, much housing renewal has occurred, promoted largely by housing associations and housing cooperatives. But unemployment is still high and poverty is rife: 80% of school children qualify for school clothing grants; that is, they come from homes with very low incomes.

Settling into Easterhouse was more difficult because we no longer had children at home and it is through children that contacts are more easily made with other families. Further, I was one of the very few English people in the area. One local punter told me, "We don't like English people here – but it's better than coming from Edinburgh". I grew to love the harsh humour. Someone else said, "Well at least you had the sense to marry a Glaswegian". I started going to the Easterhouse Salvation Army Corps which was close to our flat. This was run by a remarkable couple, Captains Eric and Ann Buchanan, who had the knack of drawing in the most needy people. Eric soon recruited me into helping at his crowded and chaotic youth clubs. I also spent time at the remains of some former shops where a few residents had set up a small cafe and a table tennis table. I often felt nervous, but my table tennis skills came in useful and won me some respect from the teenagers. Before long, I was organising clubs at the Salvation Army, was making friendships with residents and on the small committee at the shops where we started a community newspaper. However, I soon felt some hostility directed at the fact that I was funded by an external body. The other participants resented any influence from outside, so, although I was grateful to the National Children's Home, I felt it right to sever my links with them.

Poverty was extensive in Easterhouse. Yet, during these years, I began to perceive that the problem was not just poverty, it was also inequality. I met families who survived on corned beef in a society where others can spend £200 on one meal. I knew families with incomes of less than £7,000 a year in a nation where others receive over £70,000 plus extensive perks. I object to such gross inequalities and believe that God made all people of equal value so that the abundance of the earth should be shared fairly between them. I object as a socialist who knows that it is possible for government to prevent such disparities. And I object because the experience of inequality damages the well-being of many people. Professor Richard Wilkinson has shown that people at the bottom in poverty in a society such as ours, where so many are affluent, can feel alienated, excluded and worthless. Their experiences are internalised in ways which adversely affect their behaviour. Some decide, 'I give up' and react with apathy, withdrawal and anger. The outcome can be that parents do not have the energy to spend time with their children, young people lose their educational motivation, adults give up on work and many people give up on their own health. An extreme result is that some seek alternative satisfactions in drugs and crime (Wilkinson, 1994, 1996). The lesson I draw is that it is not just sufficient to alleviate poverty; it is also necessary to reduce inequalities.

I tried to add my voice to the few who still argue for a more equal society in *Towards equality* (Holman, 1997). Simultaneously, I became involved in local action. The activities I have described in the old shops finished when the builders arrived to construct new ones. A number of residents came together and founded a project called Family Action in Rogerfield and Easterhouse (FARE), with Rogerfield being our district within Easterhouse. A small grant was obtained from a charitable trust and FARE began, with no premises and myself as its part-time worker. Soon it had one room in the flat, used by the Tenants Association, and access to the use of the local primary school in the evenings. Another member of staff, Graham Hammond, was recruited. After a financial crisis in which FARE almost folded, I resigned as a paid worker but continued as a volunteer while working one day a week at Glasgow University. FARE then received coverage in two television programmes. The first was one of a series made by Central Independent Television in 1990 called 'Encounter'. The second was when Channel 4 TV set up a Commission on Poverty which went out in 1996 as 'The great, the good and the dispossessed'. FARE was one of the projects visited by the Commission. The programmes brought publicity and made it easier to get funds, and thereafter it grew. It moved into five flats which had become hard to let following some drug-related deaths within them. Today it has six staff.

What does FARE do? For children and young people, it runs extensive activities. There is a 'breakfast club' for children, particularly those whose parents have to leave for work before schools open. Youth clubs are held at lunch times in two local schools and then in the evenings in FARE's own building. The clubs benefit from the full-time leadership of Bobby Kerr, a local man who was initially drawn in when his children attended the clubs. The minibuses, driven by volunteers, are used not just for FARE's own swimming, skating and bowling trips, but also by other local groups. In the summer, holidays are organised for over a hundred children.

For the community at large, FARE has a cafe – the only one in the district – which promotes healthy eating. It has grown to the extent that a half-time cafe worker has been recruited. FARE is run on a financial shoestring, so the post is for one year, although hopefully funds will be found for three years. FARE members were involved in the establishment of a thriving credit union which now uses the building as one of its collecting points. Work with parents and young children is led by Anna McCann, who has brought up her own kids in the area, and the parents are among those who take advantage of a baby co-op, run by residents, which sells cheap nappies and baby clothes. Classes are held for those with literacy and numeracy difficulties. Expert welfare rights advice is on hand from a debt counsellor who comes in once a week.

For individuals, FARE offers friendship and counselling. The project leader, Rosemary Dickson, helps those with drug abuse problems. Matt and Diane Hall, who live a few doors from us, do a job share which includes relating with young people, often referred by the schools, who may be truanting, suspended or getting into delinquency. My own involvement has particularly been with vulnerable families.

But FARE has its limitations. It has failed to engage some residents and failed to reach some young people. It has, however, made the following contributions to the neighbourhood:

• For 11 years, it has run youth activities in a needy area. The clubs might be deemed old-fashioned, with table tennis, craft, pool, music and little in the way of expensive, modern electronic equipment. But they do draw young people into a safe environment as an alternative to being on the streets. Two 20-year-olds were asked on television why they had not got into crime and drugs. They replied that at about the age of 12, they had the option of the 'club stream' or the 'gang stream'. They chose the former (BBC 2 schools programme, 'Taking issue', 1997).

- It provides a welcoming environment to parents. Chatting in the cafe, meeting other parents, going on a family holiday, may seem insignificant to many people. But for parents under stress, who are poverty-stricken, who cannot afford holidays, such activities are important. A stressed woman clutching a baby, staggered into FARE saying that she was at the end of her tether. Volunteers looked after the baby and gave her something to eat. She felt welcomed, not judged. She was then able to tell the project leader that she was up to her neck in debts and was feeding a family of five on £30 a week.
- It responds quickly to crises. A mother, who had been on Income Support long-term, reached breaking point. FARE was almost immediately able to get her away on holiday and arrange care for her children. A lone mother was distraught when, following an argument, her son ran away. A member of staff, who knew the boy well, quickly searched for and found him. A lone parent in rent arrears experienced a chip pan fire which destroyed her cooker and some furniture. It seemed the last straw. Volunteers cleaned the mess and FARE arranged a grant to replace the cooker. The project leader began to work with the woman to address the rent arrears. She said, "At last, there is light at the end of the tunnel". Such actions can be taken without an appointment and by staff well known to, and trusted by, those in need of help.
- It provides opportunities for individuals. Carol, for example, had experienced a traumatic childhood and become a volatile single mother. While she was in a psychiatric unit, the authorities removed her daughter and later said the child would be adopted. Carol then became a volunteer at FARE and, when elected chair of one of its activities, said it was the first time she had ever been shown respect. Her self-confidence was boosted. She began to relate with other people. FARE's staff went with her to a Children's Hearing and, in the end, she regained the care of her daughter, was able to form a stable marriage, and is now a well-known local activist. Another young person, Brian, was brought up in a low-income family and found an outlet for his aggression in FARE's clubs and sports, but he seemed destined for grotty jobs and an uncertain future. Aged 19, he was taken on by FARE as a full-time young youth worker which included attending college to study sport. He is about to leave FARE after three years and hopes to pursue a career in the sports industry.

If FARE has made a significant contribution to the area, then I think it stems from the fact that it is rooted in the neighbourhood. The project is genuinely locally controlled, with committee members elected at an annual general meeting open to residents. Betty McPherson continued as an able chair from FARE's beginnings until her death in 2000, when she was succeeded by Jim Hughes. It is residents – not powerful outsiders – who decide on policies, set the budget and appoint staff. Consequently, its activities are relevant to local people because they are a response to what residents want. It is not just the committee who are local; staff, sessional workers and volunteers are also predominantly from the area. This means that they are well known, that they are regarded as neighbours, that they are available, and that staff salaries are spent within the local economy.

FARE is just one of thousands of what I call 'neighbourhood groups', which I define as the residents of a small locality acting together in projects for the collective well-being of their neighbourhood. Having visited a number of these groups and read about many more, I believe they are important for four reasons.

First, they strengthen neighbourhoods. They have recruited local volunteers, drawn in resources, started activities which were not there before and created a more positive image of their area. In short, they facilitate the self-help and the readiness to help each other which are the essence of a good neighbourhood.

Second, they are preventative. Neighbourhood groups cannot eradicate poverty, but they do provide practical services through credit unions, food co-ops, and furniture stores, which can alleviate material social deprivations and so reduce family stress. Youth clubs, sports teams and holidays can divert some young people away from unacceptable behaviour. Trusted staff, who have been in the area for years, can offer 'resourceful friendship' and counselling to adults and young people facing personal problems. As Gibbons concluded in her study of prevention, "parents under stress more easily overcome family problems ... when there are many sources of family support available in local communities" (Gibbons et al, 1990, p 162). Neighbourhood groups can thus help families stay together and reduce the number of young people accommodated in public care or sent into custody.

Third, they enable local voices to be heard. Poor people are often dismissed as unable to speak or write about social problems and policy. The truth is that they are rarely given an opportunity to express themselves in newspapers, on the radio, or on television. Notably, when New Labour set up a Social Exclusion Unit, its membership contained no poor people and no residents from the most deprived areas. Neighbourhood groups are now taking the initiative. Seven low-income Easterhouse people contributed to the book *Faith in the Poor*. They demonstrated that not only could they write movingly about their experiences, but could also suggest means of change. One big publisher turned down the book on the grounds that nobody would be interested in what the poor said. Instead, it sold out as a hardback and rapidly became a paperback (Holman, Carol, Bill, Erica, Anita, Denise, Penny and Cynthia, 1998).

Finally, the groups express important values. Of course, neighbourhood work can be beset by arguments and rivalries. But my observation is that such deficiencies are far outweighed by the constructive commitment of participants. Neighbourhood groups show that services can be provided by cooperation rather than by competition. Volunteers may well work hard for no material gain. Staff take modest salaries and tend to stay long-term rather than seeking promotion in large agencies. The groups are essentially mutual; that is, participants accept obligations towards others in the expectation that they will cooperate in building a neighbourhood which is better for all.

In terms of shaping social and economic life, these groups of low-income people in deprived zones are tiny compared with government agencies, private enterprise and establishment think-tanks. Yet they are not irrelevant to the structural causes of poverty and inequality. Ultimately, all policies spring from values. Neighbourhood groups give expression to beliefs in cooperation, equality and mutuality which would have to become widespread if income, wealth and power were ever to be redistributed. The hope must be that – in conjunction with others – the whisper from the bottom is eventually heard above those who can shout from the top.

Neighbourhood groups can attract volunteers, win the cooperation of schools and social workers, run services and handle budgets. Their major problem is that of funding. Central government will pour millions of pounds into regeneration and social inclusion partnerships dominated by professionals yet refuses to devise a strategy to provide long-term financial support to neighbourhood groups. Local authorities now place lucrative contracts with national voluntary and private agencies, yet show little enthusiasm for locals who are committed to serving and staying in their neighbourhoods. FARE, for instance, does not receive any funding from Glasgow City Council towards the salaries of its staff. Consequently, the committee of FARE is constantly engaged in raising money from charities and local fundraising activities just to survive. It is to the credit of some charitable trusts, such as the Cadbury Trust, the Lankelly Foundation and the Tudor Trust, that they are prepared to give priority to those in poverty.

Looking back, my life has revolved around family, Christianity, politics, social work and local action. After 39 years as a Labour Party activist, I have some disappointment with New Labour. I acknowledge that it has launched a multitude of policies, programmes and initiatives. The trouble is that ministers and advisors rarely live alongside poor people. As I have argued elsewhere, the new policies do not necessarily take people out of poverty (Holman, 1999). Above all, I am dismayed that New Labour has abandoned the pursuit of equality. Most tellingly, among the long list of objectives in the government paper *Opportunity for all*, no target is set concerning the reduction of the gaps between the richest and the poorest (Secretary of State for Social Security, 1999).

A New Labour which refuses both to set a decent income level and to take action against the huge material and social disparities which inevitably spring from the free market system, will never achieve socialism. But I refuse to leave the Labour Party. It is my party as much as Tony Blair's and I will endeavour to change it from within. If I have lost faith in many politicians, I have not lost faith in socialism. I believe that the political pursuit of equality, fellowship and democracy are the basics for a just, fair and happy society. I also believe that socialism is more than politics and I rejoice that there are still people whose socialism is expressed in their daily behaviour and who, in short, are servants to society.

Serving people was supremely displayed in the life of Jesus. In Christianity I find strength, comfort, values and a faith that goes beyond death for it is about a personal relationship between individuals and God. I have just reached the exact age at which my father died: 64 and a quarter. Interestingly, I had a dream in which he welcomes me into the next life. But Christianity – like many religions – is also collective, and it is about the kind of society I believe should be attained on this earth. After my early years of religious searching, alienation and failure, I am happy to be a believer in Jesus' teachings.

I am happy to be a part of the neighbourhood of Easterhouse. It is true that I have been criticised by local people – rightly so – robbed, even threatened with a meat cleaver. Much more I have found humour, compassion, mutuality and closer friendships than anywhere else. The experience of being involved with the group of people who have succeeded, against the odds, in establishing FARE has been a landmark in my life.

Annette now works for Quarriers, a voluntary agency for children and adults, formerly Quarriers Homes, and finds great satisfaction in so doing. She is highly regarded for her skills both within and without the organisation. Ever modest, she will be annoyed with me for saying so. She has been amazingly tolerant of and supportive of me, financially and emotionally. She was also supportive of our son David when he did his PhD, challenging his jargon and questioning what he was saying. David is long settled in his beloved Manchester and is a research fellow in occupational psychology. Ruth is a gynaecologist, married to Bruce, a lovely New Zealander. They have a son, Lucas, and nothing gives me more joy than to be with my grandson.

Recently, an old friend in London asked whether I really liked living in wet Glasgow. I replied that I loved it. My only dislike is the Ceilidh, the Scottish dance, held at every conceivable gathering, at which spirited Scots drag you out to the floor. For a tone-deaf "zombie", this is agony. My friend then implied that I had made a mistake in not opting to be a top academic in London where I could influence the establishment. Certainly the causes which I have supported – preserving a child care specialism, prevention, protecting private foster children, promoting greater equality – have not been marked by success. But I know my presence in London would not have made any difference. I believe that here in Easterhouse I have been able to have long-term friendships with some vulnerable families and I would not change that for anything.

My life is a contented one. Two days a week I am a volunteer with FARE; two days I look after our grandson. One day I earn some money by writing. My words are not always well received. Commenting on one of my books, Robert Whelan of the Institute of Economic Affairs, slated me as "Professor Errant" because of my "unwillingness to confront the moral failings of the poor who surround [me]" (Whelan, 1996, p 79). I must add that later we met and became good friends despite our continuing differences. What I do hope is that my writing is informed by the residents with whom I mix. I would say that I am no children's champion but I think I have one thing in common with the six others in this book: no regrets.

EIGHT

Past, present and future

The champions for children who I have described are all aged over 65 or are deceased. The book might, therefore, be dismissed as irrelevant to contemporary child care. On the contrary, the lives of the six children's champions are worth preserving in print in recognition of the enormous contribution they have made to the well-being of children. In addition, their practices, values, policies and writings have lessons for the present and the future. But the book is not only about them. It also draws on the experiences of those usually regarded just as recipients of services or as residents of deprived areas. They too have much to teach.

A family service

Four of the six child care champions were closely involved with the local authority Children's Departments. Marjory Allen headed up the campaign which brought about their creation. Barbara Kahan was a successful children's officer who pioneered preventative work. John Stroud established that children in care ideally needed contact with their natural families. Clare Winnicott defined child care casework and organised the training of child care officers who specialised in relating to deprived children. Although Children's Departments had many weaknesses, nonetheless, considering that they existed for less than 25 years, their achievements were remarkable.

The Children's Departments were amalgamated into the social services departments (SSDs) in England and Wales and the social work departments (SWDs) in Scotland. Beyond doubt, the new service led to improvements for user groups which were previously neglected, particularly older people. Within the child and family sphere, important improvements have followed regarding juvenile justice and child protection. Certainly the much larger SSDs became equal to other leading local authority services such as Education Departments, possessed increased political influence and, for a while, won large increases in budgets. But there is a strongly held viewpoint – one with which I agree – that child care standards have declined. Barbara Kahan has long identified this decline. Professor Roy Parker has written,

"There is clearly a need for social workers to acquire more skill in direct work with children.... This has to be remedied if children's views are to be elicited; if they are to understand their past and present situations; and if they are to be encouraged to fulfil their potential" (Parker, 1999, p 112). Professor Jane Tunstill, another articulate child care campaigner, has highlighted the decline of prevention (Tunstill, 1999).

The deterioration in child care practice appears to have stemmed from the following factors. First, SSDs and SWDs have become multi-service agencies. Not only were they an amalgamation of various services but, from 1971, many more duties in regard to child care, disabled and older people were thrust on them. Lady Allen's objective of an organisation which could concentrate on deprived children was abandoned. In terms of resources, child care often lost out in competition with other user groupings. Moreover, as cuts were imposed on the child care sections, it was frequently residential establishments which bore the brunt – with disastrous results, as Barbara Kahan made clear.

Second, in the years following reorganisation, many of the new departments went 'generic', meaning that social workers dealt with a whole range of different client types.

When the shortcomings of this approach became clear, most departments set up child care sections within the SSDs and SWDs. But, by this time, specialist child care skills had declined and, as older staff retired, there was a lack of specialists in senior, supervisory and teaching posts.

Third, as social work training also went generic so, to cite what Barbara Kahan has written,

> ... it was possible to qualify as a social worker having spent only a few sessions in two years on any matters related to child care. In relation to the complexity and delicacy of many issues affecting children and young people, with implications not only for their immediate present but for many years of their later lives, it is unnecessary to spell out some of the consequences of such gaps in knowledge and skills on the part of staff responsible for analysis, support and decision making on their behalf. (Kahan, 1999)

Fourth, the new departments became very bureaucratic. Bureaucracy can be a force for efficiency or inefficiency. Within the 'Seebohm factories', as they were known, the complex administrative systems and layers of management became, as Jane Packman put it, a source of "misdirection, distortion and loss of a sense of urgency...." (Packman, 1975, p 171). A report on the death of a child on an 'at-risk' register noted the low morale of staff in a large department, their lack of child care skills, and poor communication with other agencies (Bridge Child Care Development Service, 1997). Onerous procedures, form filling and meetings so absorbed social workers that they had less time for a personal approach with children and for links with other services.

Finally, child care itself became dominated by issues of child abuse and the doctrine of permanency. From the time of the inquiry into the tragic death of Maria Colwell in 1973, SSDs and SWDs moved to protect themselves from criticisms in the media that they were leaving children in the care of dangerous parents (DHSS, 1974b). In a sense, child protection became a specialism as resources were poured into child protection teams, manuals and training. As David Thorpe concluded from his study, "The new ideology appears to have succeeded in changing the role of child welfare agencies from one of service provision, to one of policing" (Thorpe, 1994, p 199). More recently, Professor Chris Jones, in a study of experienced social workers, observes that now "traditional, mainstream client focussed social work has little place in current state social work agencies" (Jones, 2001). In this climate, it has become difficult for social workers to be 'resourceful friends' or to relate to children in the way that child care officers had done.

Of course, prevention and personal child care did not disappear. Following the publication of the Barclay Report in 1982, what was called 'community social work' enjoyed a brief summer as some social workers worked closely alongside the residents of deprived estates (NISW, 1982). The 1989 Children Act and the 1995 Children Act (Scotland) gave approval both to protection and to family support. Skilled child care staff still exist. But they are often working against the odds. People in need cannot be sure of finding the kind of skilled and personal social work help of yesteryear.

The present position has been powerfully expressed in a letter to *Community Care*. The author stated:

> As part of the work I do I come into contact with families who are unhappy with the service they have received from their local social services department. Almost without fail those families identify that their experience is one of not being listened to, not being understood and not being treated with simple respect and kindness. They say social workers seem to have an agenda that does not have the family's anxieties nor the welfare of their children as its starting point. (Brand, 1999)

The writer generalises but there is much in what she says. It is not that social workers lack compassion or concern; rather – unlike child care officers – they function within structures which push them into acting as monitors, assessors and what are sometimes called 'soft policemen'.

What can be done to improve child care social work? My proposal is for the formation of new local authority Family Departments. They would take over responsibilities for vulnerable children from SSDs and SWDs while new adult SWDs would accept their other duties. I would also give the new Family Departments responsibility for youth services (often called youth and community services in Scotland) on the grounds that youth work activities can often play an important part in improving life for young people. The objectives of this family service would be as follows:

- to promote the welfare of children and young people in need, if possible within their own families;
- to prevent the ill-treatment and abuse of children and young people;
- to encourage them not to commit offences against the law;
- to provide high quality services from skilled child care social workers (or family workers as I will now call them) who relate with the young people and their families, often in conjunction with substitute carers in foster or adoptive families or trained staff in residential establishments.

Structures and objectives are necessary, but alone they are not sufficient. I am a football fanatic and I know that the sport could not function without the ordinances which determine the numbers of players in the teams and the rules of play. In addition, teams have to apply tactics, methods and ploys which can be called 'approaches to the game'. In like manner, Family Departments must have structures and duties prescribed by legislation. But success will also depend on the approaches they adopt in order to achieve objectives. I see two as crucial.

One is a family orientation. In its document *Supporting families*, the present Labour government argues that families are the bedrock of society (Home Office, 1998). In keeping with this, Family Departments would strive to ensure not only that, where possible, children stay with their own families but also that all families enjoy the social supports which encourage – rather than undermine – good parenting. To this end, the departments would be able to offer day care, family aides, home helps and other supportive services. These would be coordinated by trained family workers able to exercise the kind of skills, knowledge, values and commitment taught by Clare Winnicott, promoted by Barbara Kahan and practised by John Stroud. These include the ability to help parents understand their difficulties along with the warm encouragement that can enable them to persist through these difficulties. When children and young people do have to leave home, these skills can be employed by family workers to communicate sensitively with these children to explain what is happening, to prepare them for the next steps, and to maintain positive links with home.

The other crucial approach is through a community emphasis. Removals into public care, delinquency, child abuse and other social malaises are not confined to, but are more concentrated in, socially deprived neighbourhoods. These same neighbourhoods are often the children's familiar ground, the location of their schools and clubs and the source of friends and relatives. It makes sense for teams of family workers and their colleagues to be based within small and neglected neighbourhoods. Their location would make them known to and closer to families, increase their understanding of local dynamics and improve liaison with other services.

In addition, the teams would have more opportunities for improving community life. Family Departments would have the responsibility to provide youth facilities which can be so important to young people who are often distanced from leisure amenities. These facilities, open to all young people, would serve to bolster the positive image of departments as serving the whole community, not just those who are stigmatised with the titles of 'delinquents', 'drug abusers' and 'trouble makers'.

In the previous chapter, I stressed the value of projects, like the Southdown Project, whose strengths spring from staff living long-term in the areas, developing 'resourceful friendships' and involving residents. Statutory departments may face difficulties in directly running similar agencies. Family workers, as well as using preventative measures, would still investigate suspected abuse and, where necessary, take steps to remove children. These actions might well create tensions with some residents which would make it difficult for staff to reside alongside them. Further, statutory workers are often on career ladders which entail them moving on after two or three years. I believe that the national voluntary child care societies, of which little has been said in this book, could have a role here. Despite their pioneering beginnings, in recent years they have become closely associated with local authorities and often receive large contracts to help them carry out their statutory duties. If the voluntaries took on the role of funding their staff to live and stay long-term in deprived areas, they would again be providing something different from local authorities.

In a later section, I will say more about the funding of local, independent neighbourhood groups.

The proposal for Family Departments is a radical one which goes against current trends for extending management, for less specialisation and for more amalgamation of services. In November 1999, Hertfordshire announced it would merge its SSDs and its educational services. A year later, the council of Rhondda Cynon Taff in Wales announced it was shifting services for deprived and needy children into a new Education and Lifelong Learning Department. Others have merged SSDs or SWDs with housing services. Now the government is carrying through legislation to allow the creation of Health and Social Care Trusts. Social work services for adults seem certain to be drawn into these huge bodies. The SSDs' and SWDs' children's services will either join them or be hived off to Education Departments. If this happens, not only is a child care specialism further undermined, but the very occupation of social work is endangered. In the present culture, which favours huge empires dominated by managers rather than by social workers, the proposal for Family Departments will incur the criticism that they would be too small to be effective. I am not arguing for a return to Children's Departments, but rather for Family Departments which would be larger than the former Children's Departments yet smaller than SSDs and SWDs. Interestingly, a study of Nordic countries points out that their children's services are small compared with British ones but have high child care standards, effective communication with other bodies and are well regarded by the populace (Cohen and Rea Price, 1996).

Without denying that Family Departments would have limitations, I believe these would be outweighed by the following advantages:

- *A clear focus*: Family Departments would have the singular aim of improving the family life of children. Unlike the multi-aim and complex SSDs and SWDs (and whatever replaces them), this focus would be understood not only by staff and users but also by the public at large.
- *Moderate size*: unity of purpose and a sense of mission are easier to cultivate in services where members know and see each other. In Family Departments, managers would be less distant, hierarchies less onerous and paperwork less complex. With more time, family workers could pursue the close and personal relationships with users which were an attribute of many Children's Departments.
- *Specialism*: an agency which focuses just on children and their parents would develop specialised skills. Unlike the Children's Departments,

these would be practised frequently within the context of neighbourhoods.

* *Family support*: a commitment to family life, family workers equipped with preventative skills, supportive services, a community approach, the provision of youth facilities and local voluntary projects would all combine to strengthen families. It would enable more vulnerable parents to cope with their children and improve the general quality of family life within deprived locations. The emphasis on family support need not entail the neglect of children at risk of child abuse. The evidence suggests that locally-based staff who know and become known in neighbourhoods not only spot potential abuse at an early stage, but are able to offer effective help (Holman, 1993, pp 75-6).

A National Neighbourhood Fund

Local authority Family Departments could strengthen the areas where families are most vulnerable to disruption and social deprivations. But their services would not be sufficient alone. My experience in Easterhouse led me to identify some of the benefits to such areas from locally run community projects or, as they are sometimes called, neighbourhood groups. Bill Jordan is one of the foremost experts on social work and he regrets that its emphasis on relationships is being undermined by a social work which is mechanistic and monitory. Yet he sees hope in the emergence of projects "which are between the formal world of the local authorities, the big voluntary agencies and the commercial sector, and the everyday world of citizens' lives" (Jordan, 2000, p 207). He is referring partly to neighbourhood groups. Unfortunately, they are chronically underfunded. Central government refuses directly to finance local projects. Local authorities are increasingly using their voluntary budgets to fund the national charities which are large enough to take over certain local government duties and therefore have fewer resources available for local projects. Local activists had hoped that the government's much publicised neighbourhood renewal programme would award a leading role to neighbourhood projects. Instead, its strategy document reveals that partnerships of large organisations will take the lead, along with the money and the power. Local residents and their groups will be able to apply for funds from community chests, but only lip service is paid to their role. The amounts available are peanuts; overall just a fraction of the £250 million of public money spent on

Portcullis House which provides luxury offices for MPs (Social Exclusion Unit, 2001).

My proposal is for a government-funded National Neighbourhood Fund. It would distribute money to local Neighbourhood Trusts in the most severely deprived areas (the government numbers them at 3,000) and in turn the trusts would allocate grants to locally controlled neighbourhood groups and projects. Residents would elect members of their neighbourhood trusts while the latter would elect the members of the central National Neighbourhood Fund. The outcomes would be as follows:

- an extension of democracy: the kind of people usually excluded from power gain places on bodies able to distribute resources;
- an increase in employment: credit unions, food co-ops, youth projects and so on afford more staff. Moreover, being local staff, they would spend their salaries within their districts and so boost the local economy;
- a multiplication of low-income residents involved as committee members, volunteers and staff in neighbourhood projects. They would not only contribute to community activities, also they personally would benefit as their confidence is lifted;
- a growth and improvement in local services, the services which residents want, the services which can improve the quality of family and neighbourhood life. These services play a vital part in helping parents to cope with their children and in diverting young people away from trouble.

A more equal society

The government's own figures (ONS, 1998, pp 9-13, 1999, ch 5) demonstrate that poverty and gross inequality continue in Britain. Poverty and inequality harm their victims socially, educationally, physically and emotionally. Professor David Donnison writes, "Since profoundly unequal societies recreate poverty and its hardships in new forms in every generation, the drive to lift every citizen out of poverty cannot succeed unless it becomes a drive for greater equality" (Donnison, 2001, p 22).

Figures are essential. In addition, I am moved daily by meeting people in poverty who suffer because of societal inequality. Our project, FARE, received a modest hardship fund from the Charities Advisory Trust to help residents in desperate need. To date, three kinds of grants have gone to 50 families. For 27 families, grants were for emergencies, such as for a lone mother who was penniless for four days after she was mugged. For 14 families, grants were for unanticipated events, such as when a low-income parent received an enormous funeral bill after her teenage son was stabbed to death. For nine families, grants were for basic domestic items with, for example, a washing machine being provided for an unemployed widow supporting four young people. All but three of the families depended on Income Support, with the majority in receipt of a Social Fund loan from the Benefits Agency. These loans are repaid by automatic deductions so the weekly incomes of families were between £5 and £15 less even than the government's calculation of the minimum on which families can survive. As their plight worsened, some families then also turned to high interest credit companies for cookers, clothes and furniture. One shop in Easterhouse draws in poor families by promising no credit investigations and immediate delivery. The catch is an extremely high interest rate which means that purchasers end up paying double the cash price. A few days ago a catalogue came through our letter box from a cheque company offering '£100 for you to spend right now'. The APR over 25 weeks was 152%. This type of borrowing can result in situations like that of a lone parent who I know well, whose weekly income was £113.88 with a total expenditure – including debt repayments – of £113.25. It was impossible to save, and when she bought some Christmas presents she fell behind on repayments and was about to have her bed and cooker repossessed until FARE's hardship fund was used to help her.

New Labour has brought about improvements with increased child benefit, a minimum wage and the Working Families' Tax Credit. But it refuses to state just what the income is for a decent lifestyle. In the 1930s, Eleanor Rathbone's pleas to government to detail the costs of a minimum living standard fell on deaf ears. The ears are still not listening. Significantly, when the Family Budget Unit of London University worked out, in precise detail, the cost of "a low cost but acceptable lifestyle", its incomes were well above those given on Income Support and minimum wages (Parker, 1998, p 88).

I constantly observe inequality. Ours is a society in which, in 1998-99, many citizens had incomes of over £50,000 a year, the kind of incomes which allow for very comfortable lifestyles (ONS, 1999, Table 5.3, p 93). Yet I have recently come across the following:

> *On a freezing December evening, I visit a family who cannot afford a can of calor gas for the fire in their damp flat.*

Our project runs cheap holidays yet it still has to subsidise some kids for a week camping in a wet field.

I lent a few 'quid' to a family who had just one pound left for the weekend. A pound is not sufficient for a power card to provide heat, not enough to get food for their children. The parents were reluctant to ask for a 'tap' from me but were forced on by their worries for their children.

Poverty and inequality of this kind are simply not acceptable. I long for the abolition of poverty. I want a more equal society. By this I do not mean a society in which everyone is identical to each other. Rather, I mean a society in which resources, opportunities and responsibilities are so distributed as not to place any individuals or sections of the population at severe social or material disadvantage compared with others. In the first decade of the 20th century, Eleanor Rathbone perceived that charity and social work could not counter poverty. Family Departments and a National Neighbourhood Fund, which I advocate, can do much to improve the lives of children, parents and communities but they cannot provide all people with decent incomes or erase inequality. What reforms are required to counter these problems? In Chapter Six, the reforms recommended by Peter Townsend were highlighted. Here let me draw on the recommendations of an economist for whom I have much respect. Will Hutton initially made his mark as a London stockbroker. If he had stayed in the city, he was assured of an enormous income and lucrative positions in financial institutions and private companies. Instead, he opted for journalism where his brilliant newspaper columns identified the stark inequalities which inevitably flow from the free market. Once New Labour was in power, Hutton might have obtained highly paid government sinecures and a seat in the House of Lords if he had chosen to ingratiate himself with the establishment. Instead, he continued his radical attacks on New Labour's failure to promote greater equality. His proposals include the following:

- *Progressive taxation*: he calls for a system of direct taxation which would "address the incomes and privileges of the rich"(Hutton, 2000, p 22), in particular, increased income, inheritance and property taxes. He estimates that such taxes would bring in about £5 billion a year which could be used for the benefit of others.
- *Maximum income*: Hutton wants a regulatory force to determine and limit the pay levels of those 'at the top'.

- *Countering poverty*: he writes, "There needs to be a big boost in the incomes of the poor. British Income Support is extraordinarily mean" (Hutton, 2000, p 23).
- *Educational change*: Hutton argues that state schools must be improved so as to develop the potential of every child. He adds, "In the meantime, the charitable status of private schools should be withdrawn.... Selection procedures for university should be biased in favour of poorer kids in order to redress some of the advantages conferred by birth into richer homes" (Hutton, 2000, p 24).
- *Employment improvements*: he advocates restructuring industry in order to create better paid, more secure careers rather than low-paid, insecure jobs.

Relate, activate, agitate

Hutton's proposals are not exhaustive but they are on the right track in that they would both counter poverty and also promote greater financial and social equality.

Proposals to abolish poverty and diminish inequality always meet the objection – often from those with high incomes and high status – that the economy could not afford such expenditure. In the late 1940s, a Labour government made Britain's most radical social changes of the 20th century and did so at a time when the economy was still drained by the costs of war. Fifty years later, the economy is in its healthiest state for years. Redistribution of resources is possible.

Britain could afford massively to reduce social deprivations. Felicity Lawrence reports that Britain now has 74,000 millionaires with the number increasing by 17% a year. It is a country with numerous people who have well-paid jobs plus high incomes from directorships and investments, with people whose income and wealth far exceed their needs (Lawrence, 2001). The wealthy, the politicians and the establishment – or what Jeremy Paxman calls the 'establishments' (Paxman, 1991) – are not genuinely in favour of the changes that could transform the lives of the poor of this country. Does this mean reform is impossible? Not at all. When Eleanor Rathbone was young, the idea of family allowances was not even discussed. By the time of her death, they were on the statute book. When Peter Townsend was born, the Poor Law was still in existence, unemployment was widespread, access to proper medical care was the preserve of those in secure jobs and poor children could rarely proceed to higher education. By the 1950s, the Poor Law had been abolished, unemployment was low, the NHS was in operation and Peter was among the first generation of working-class young people to be given free university education. When Marjory Allen was at school, the prospect of a local authority department with a brief to give personal care to deprived children was not considered. Her determined campaigning contributed to the establishment of Children's Departments. Change is possible. But it must start with us. We are the people who can influence politics. We must continually voice the values that show that poverty in the midst of riches is incompatible with a humane society. Members of political parties must challenge the absence of the subject of inequality from the political agenda. As individuals, we can, by our own lifestyles, reveal a willingness to take no more than the average income and to participate with 'excluded' people in agitating for a better, fairer society. In short, we can relate, activate and agitate. A thousand small matches can make a powerful blaze. Change is possible.

Champions for children

This book is mainly about six champions for children. So, at its close, it is appropriate to return to them. Eleanor Rathbone again and again argued that every family should have the right to a decent income. Marjory Allen made the case for a local authority service which concentrated just on deprived children. Barbara Kahan demonstrated how that service could become a reality. John Stroud – with emotion and humour – showed that all parents are important to their children and that services should aim to prevent family disruptions. Clare Winnicott equipped hundreds of students to provide a personal and skilled service to children. Peter Townsend has tirelessly campaigned against all kinds of poverty, but particularly child poverty.

People today would do well to learn from the achievements of the champions for they have contributed to the well-being of children, particularly the most vulnerable children in our society. And lessons can be learnt not just from their achievements but also from their characters and approaches. They were driven more by a cause than by a career. Eleanor Rathbone could have used her enormous talents to become a cabinet minister if she had joined a major political party. She opted to remain an independent so as to be free to pursue her passion for social justice. Marjory Allen did become a 'Lady' when her husband was ennobled. But it seemed not to matter to her and she always regretted that they lost old friends who considered that his acceptance of a peerage was in contradiction to his earlier principles. Her major cause, pursued with passion, became the foundation of a system of child care that really met the needs of deprived children. Barbara Kahan did not – as is common today – hop from top post to top post in search of ever-higher salaries and power. Her dedication was seen in her staying with the same Children's Department for 20 years. John Stroud served even longer with another department. He did so not to gain recognition from the establishment, on the contrary he kept his distance from those at the top. He was fired by compassion for the kind of children he described in his novels. Clare Winnicott was dedicated to inspiring child care officers. She put this before her academic career and before writing books. Peter Townsend has put the cause of poor people before his own self-advancement.

Another lesson that can be learnt from these champions is that they were willing to be unpopular for the sake of the cause. Eleanor Rathbone endured many snipes and initially received little support for her proposal that women receive an allowance independent of their husbands. She persisted in her campaign for most of her life. Marjory Allen, in criticising standards of child care in the 1940s, caused great offence. She was accused of wanting to destroy the voluntary sector and even of using child care as a means of making money by her own writings. In fact, she died with little money but could be considered rich in what she had achieved for children. Barbara Kahan's determination to provide delinquent young people with something better than approved schools increased the expenditure of her department. The result was conflict with officials and councillors. The battles almost certainly cost her the post of director of social services when the Children's Departments were abolished. John Stroud's early determination to reunite children with long-lost parents sometimes annoyed older figures who considered that 'failed' parents were a bad influence. Peter Townsend has been prepared to be unpopular with the Labour Party of which he is a member and to receive the vitriol of newspapers in his determination to show that poverty is not being fully countered in Britain. In short, these champions have put the interests of needy families before self-interest. Today, more than ever, we need people like them in order to achieve a better deal for children who are vulnerable to separation, isolation, unhappiness, delinquency and social deprivations.

I have learnt much from these child care champions. Many of my values and practices have been shaped by them. I have also come to know, love and learn from others who are not regarded as experts. On council estates I have encountered criminals, child abusers, drug dealers

Epilogue

Champions for children appeared in 2001. With the death of Peter Townsend in 2009 all the champions discussed in this book are now dead. But they are not forgotten. Eleanor Rathbone's contribution has been articulated in recent debates about child benefit while Frank Field MP continues to draw attention to her distinguished parliamentary career. Marjory Allen's name is still attached to old and new adventure playgrounds. Barbara Kahan is known to today's social workers for her careful analysis of what is required from children's residential care and for her success in drawing attention to child abuse. John Stroud's novels, particularly *The shorn lamb*, still sell, and his bringing together of literature and childcare has been praised in an academic journal (see Hardy, 2005). A biography of Clare Winnicott was published in 2004 which led to renewed interest in the part she played in supporting her husband, the child psychiatrist, Donald Winnicott, as well as her expertise as a psychoanalyst (Kanter, 2004). Peter Townsend was amazingly prolific, both as a researcher and writer, right up until his death. Since then, his writings have continued to be read widely, with his life celebrated in *The Peter Townsend reader*, including contributions from a number of academic experts (Walker et al, 2010).

There is something more. The social conditions, the nature of social services agencies and the financial circumstances of the families who were the concern of these champions have changed significantly in recent years. The question arises: are the champions still relevant? I believe they are, but limit myself to just one aspect of each of them in which I think we can still learn from them.

Eleanor Rathbone

The economic crash of 2009-10 in Britain was caused by bankers and financers making too many loans at high interest that could not be re-paid. In the midst came the election of a Coalition government (Conservatives and Liberal Democrats), whose austerity policies involving huge cuts in public spending have led to greater unemployment, frozen wages at the lower end, fixed social benefits and less effective social services. In turn, these policies have contributed to a huge drop in the incomes and living conditions of thousands of families.

The official measure of poverty remains at those in households with incomes below 60% of the median income. By 2011, 3.8 million children were living in poverty, with the Child Poverty Action Group (CPAG) calculating that this would increase by another 600,000 by 2013 (CPAG, 2011). Even though the minimum wage was raised in 2011 to £6.08 an hour, research at Loughborough University has demonstrated that this will not be sufficient to provide the necessities of life, and recommend an increase to £7.20 an hour. Yet 20% of employees were earning less than this amount (Stewart, 2011).

Low incomes and benefits have led to increased homelessness that has made it even harder for some parents to cope with their children. The Trussell Trust, which provides food parcels to families who receive a voucher from social workers or other officials, expanded its number of branches rapidly in 2012. A survey of teachers in the same year recorded that 83% had seen pupils coming into school hungry (Campbell and Butler, 2012).

The response of government ministers to the growth in poverty and unemployment has been three-fold. First, Prime Minister David Cameron called for parenting groups to train parents in how to look after their children properly and, in particular, to equip them with the skills and motivations to succeed at school and to obtain jobs. Second, the Department for Work and Pensions contracted with mainly private firms to ensure that unemployed people – including many disabled people – sought and obtained employment. And third, severe pressure and punishments have been applied to the workless in the form of having to work without pay or having benefits reduced.

Iain Duncan Smith, currently Secretary of State for Work and Pensions, displayed some compassion towards those in poverty while he was in Opposition, but this changed when he came to office. In 2012 he declared, 'If you just give people money, they almost always just feed the problem, such as drug addiction, you don't solve it' (*The Guardian*, 2012). A few months later, *The Observer* reported on a paper by The Centre of Social Justice, founded by Iain Duncan Smith, and said that 'It was unremitting in its determination to frame child poverty as mainly an issue of morality and behaviour, citing adult addiction, poor parenting, worklessness and family breakdown' as the cause (*The Observer*, 2012). Government ministers and the right-wing press blamed 'lazy adults' for preferring to live off benefits rather than work. These 'lazy adults' then ended up raising children who copied their bad habits.

The solution was to push them into jobs, through private firms, with little regard for their health or the low wages they might receive. Those, especially the young, who did not try hard enough to find work would have their benefits reduced or even removed. From April 2012, 124,000 unemployed single parents with children about to start school were instructed to find work within eight weeks or risk losing benefits. Parents were not allowed to choose to stay with their young children if they thought this the best way to maintain family life and healthy parent–child relationships. The imposition of a housing benefit cap means that numbers are now being forced to move to areas with cheaper rents despite the adverse effect this has on making children change schools and friendships and despite the fact that the areas are more likely to have high unemployment. In June 2012, the Prime Minister announced that he intended to scrap housing benefit for those aged under 25 living in council or private rented housing. He said, 'The system is saying to these people. Can't afford a home of your own? Tough, live with your parents.' He added that those who did not find work after two years on Jobseeker's Allowance would face compulsory community work (*The Herald*, 2012b).

Eleanor Rathbone's relevance is that she too lived in times when many were in deep poverty, when they were blamed for their low incomes, and were punished by the harsh Poor Law. On re-reading information about her, I was impressed again by three factors that counter those of the present government. First, in a study of casual labourers, she emphasised the strengths of poor mothers despite the erratic employment of their husbands. Some mothers pooled resources to run money clubs that enabled them to overcome fluctuations in their incomes. Second, she recorded the low wages of many male workers that was not due to their lack of willingness to work hard. Third, she perceived how the state, through the Poor Law, tended to blame and punish the poor. She acknowledged that although a minority of women were negligent and immoral to the detriment of their families, the majority were not, but if they became destitute, they were condemned and harassed by officials. She concluded that poverty was imposed on families by an economic system and unhelpful state policies. Her recommendation that mothers required an allowance paid direct to them came into being as Family Allowance in 1945. It was never at the financial level she wanted, and has now been weakened by Working Tax Credits that subsidise employers so that they can pay lower wages.

Eleanor's analysis can still be applied today – the poor should not be blamed for their poverty; the majority of children living in poverty have parents who are in work; and addiction occurs only among 4% of families. The Prime Minister, in saying that the under-25s should be forced to move back in with their parents, overlooked that some did not have parents and that others had parents who had no spare rooms. He has also failed to grasp that cutting benefits by millions will remove money that had been spent locally and that had maintained local shops and jobs.

Recent research has undermined the notion that Britain is impoverished by a welfare culture that many of those on benefits have chosen to follow as a lifestyle choice. The Joseph Rowntree Foundation sponsored a study, headed by Professor Tracey Shildrick, which interviewed people aged between 30 and 60 who were in low-paid jobs or on benefits. She also drew on material from 230 individuals in deprived areas. An important finding was that long-term unemployment was comparatively rare. Instead, those studied tended to move in and out of badly paid, temporary jobs and in and out of state benefits. Shildrick wrote, 'The important story of commitment to taking poor quality jobs, which often pay too little to move people away from poverty and make a real difference to their lives, runs directly counter to the dominant popular story about welfare dependency' (2012). There is little, if any, evidence of an entrenched welfare dependency. On the contrary, most sought work and, when they found it, it was usually through their own efforts and not through the privately run welfare to work firms. They were prepared to travel long and costly distances to undertake unpleasant tasks which brought them little more than if they stayed on welfare benefits.

These findings confirm my own observations while living in deprived neighbourhoods for over a quarter of a century – I know that most residents are anything but work-shy. More typical is a middle-aged friend who is long-term unemployed, but every week he applies for jobs. If he gets an interview he may be competing against a score of other applicants. He wanted to accompany a youth camp to help as a volunteer, which would have been good work experience. But he was, in my view, punished by job centre officials who refused him permission to go as it coincided with the day he was due to sign on and he was required to be available for work. And this, in a place where one advertisement for an administrative worker received over 950 applicants. I kid not. My friend has now been directed to unpaid voluntary work that mainly involves digging gardens. The fact is that many families are in poverty despite being well-living citizens and good parents. They did not bring about the recession, and they did not increase unemployment. Their poverty is mainly due to a lack of money.

What would Eleanor Rathbone's proposals be for today? Family Allowance set at a level sufficient to ensure that basic needs could be met? A level of wages that would take families out of poverty? Their income would be spent in their communities and would help revive the economy. Not least, those on lower incomes should be treated with respect and encouragement, not blame and condemnation.

Marjory Allen

In the original book, I chose Marjory Allen as a champion mainly because of her leading role in improving the care of children in public agencies. I also made mention of her interest in the need of all children to experience and enjoy play. It is this interest that I find particularly relevant today.

Play can be defined as voluntary activities in which children find recreational enjoyment. Academics regard it as making an important contribution to cognitive development and socialisation. Marjory Allen was no academic but she understood the importance of play. As a mother in the 1930s, she formed and ran a nursery school to which she took her daughter, Polly. It was more like the latter day playgroups in which children played freely with adults near at hand.

After the outbreak of the Second World War in 1939, she was concerned about mothers, evacuated with small children, who had to leave their landladies in the morning and wander around until they were allowed back in at blackout time. Marjory campaigned for nursery centres where children could play, rest and be fed. She succeeded in raising the money – and the interest of the government – to establish a number of centres.

In the cities, the Ministry of Health promoted day nurseries where working mothers could leave their children. However, the staffing of the nurseries was dominated by health professionals who, Marjory claimed, were not adept at promoting play. Anticipating that day nurseries were likely to decline after the war when there would be less demand for women workers, she campaigned for nursery schools to be mandatory for all local authorities, nursery schools that regarded play as central. Legislation to this end was passed in 1944, but its implementation was consistently postponed.

After the war, Marjory became interested in the growing number of adventure playgrounds and soon became chair of the London Adventure Playground Association. These playgrounds, usually located in the open air in urban areas, allowed children to take adventurous risks in the presence of skilled staff. The one of which I was a committee member in Handsworth, Birmingham, saw children lighting fires and cooking meals on them, climbing trees, swinging on ropes and building dens in concrete pipes. It also contained a wooden hut in which games could be played when it rained. Adventure playgrounds encourage children to play together, to care for domestic animals that may be kept on the site, to learn how to construct objects from raw materials and, above all, how to enjoy themselves in the open air.

During the early 1960s, pre-school playgroups multiplied. They are organised groups for children mostly between the ages of two and five and usually run by voluntary groups in local halls. Initially run by volunteers, in particular, parents, the formation of the Pre-school Playgroups Association became a stimulus for training the leaders, for conferences and, in some places, the payment of professional staff. I remember speaking at its annual conference that was attended by hundreds who displayed a tremendous enthusiasm for what they were doing.

The playgroups were not intended to provide full-time care for the children, with a playgroup session lasting two to three hours, and children attending two to five times a week. Parents could stay for the whole session but often just stayed until their children were settled. They were not seen as nursery schools but as places where children enjoyed play in the company of other children and under the guidance and care of interested adults. Of course, play is a means of learning, of being introduced to constructing models, becoming familiar with books, painting and singing. But there were no exams, no educational curriculum. In 1972, Sir Keith Joseph, speaking at a conference of the Pre-school Playgroups Association, identified playgroups as a major means of developing children's 'social and intellectual needs' (quoted in Butterworth and Holman, 1975, p 375).

The centrality of children's play has since declined. After the war, I spent much of my free time in a nearby park. I recall 30-a-side football matches with a tennis ball, cricket, rounders, races – all organised by ourselves. A number of adults were always strolling around. Today, far fewer children play in parks unless accompanied by parents. The reasons include a vast increase in traffic that makes crossing roads to the parks more dangerous, and a reduction in the number of supervisors we called 'the parkies'. Many parents now feel that their children are not safe on their own and could be approached by strangers. It may well be that the availability of long hours of television and electronic games give children alternative pleasures at home. Not least, statutory bodies have sold off much public ground to house builders.

From the 1990s onwards, adventure playgrounds found it increasingly difficult to obtain funding and sites. The one with which I had been associated in Birmingham folded when its ground was required for the construction of a school. The playgrounds did not disappear, however, and at least eight still include Marjory Allen's name in their title. The same applied to pre-school playgroups, the demand for which has declined as local authority and private day nurseries have been opened to cater for the children whose parent or parents were working full-time. And statutory nursery schools expanded for children aged five and under. These certainly made provision for play but were geared to prepare children for school and for climbing the educational ladder. The excellent Pre-school Playgroups Association has now disbanded.

Youth clubs have found it more difficult to obtain grants just to provide children with indoor activities that the children attended for the sheer enjoyment – grants have become linked to targets for acquiring skills or awards. I recall FARE (Family Action in Rogerfield and Easterhouse) being offered funding to get a certain number of young people off drugs. At a meeting, local parents were opposed because it was felt that it would turn the project into a centre for drug users and not one serving the whole neighbourhood, one in which parents would send their children just to play. A survey in Scotland in March 2012 found that nearly half of families could not afford a holiday. Charities like FARE run holidays that children enjoy, but just at the time when more families would like their children to be able to go, so FARE has experienced cuts in its funding. Play for its own sake is no longer considered a priority (Hamilton, 2012).

Marjory Allen's insistence on the importance of play must be revived. Public parks should again be full of children playing, although the parks would need to be supervised – not by the old 'parkies' who marched around waving walking sticks, but by a new breed of 'park prefects' capable of keeping children safe without dictating what they should play. In a small way, they could be the creation of a new occupation. Parents and grandparents should be encouraged to accompany their children and grandchildren across busy roads and be close to the smallest children on the swings and other equipment. And in one corner, there should be an adventure playground. The revival of parks could well gain the backing of a large part of the population.

Marjory did not limit herself to playgrounds, however. She regarded play as central to children's homes, groups for mothers and children, day nurseries and nursery schools. I urge central and local government and child care voluntary bodies to ensure that child play is built into all agencies that cater for children. There are signs that some authorities are stirring. In 2012 Edinburgh City Council Strategy Committee voted to ensure that all children had access to 'good outdoor play areas that help development and keep them healthy' (*The Herald*, 2012a). Unfortunately, doubts have been expressed as to whether the money can be found. And this in a local authority much criticised for enormous over-payment of staff employed to oversee the building of its city trams project – which, with rising costs, has still not been completed.

Barbara Kahan

Barbara Kahan died in August 2000. Terry Philpot wrote in an obituary, 'Across the last half century, Barbara Kahan, who has died aged 80, had a decisive effect on local authority children's departments and their successors, the all-purpose social services departments' (Philpot, 2000). The 'decisive effect' was because she was the best-known child care expert who was listened to by cabinet ministers, other MPs and top civil servants. She was also a leading member of the Association of Children's Officers that, with the Association of Child Care Officers, contributed to the shape of new legislation. She frequently featured in the press. At one point she was criticised by a right-wing newspaper as they considered her too soft on delinquents. Barbara saw it as an opportunity to answer back.

Barbara could speak as an expert on social work matters because of her own background, experiences and practice. Her father and grandfather had worked on the railways, and she knew about working-class life. When she was a girl, she had persuaded her mother to take in a Jewish refugee who stayed for her childhood. Barbara observed and understood the needs of a refugee separated from his or her own parents. Later, as a children's officer, she maintained direct contact with clients, or users, as they became known. Later in life, she kept in touch with 10 young people who had been in the care of her children's department (Kahan, 1980). She was thus able to convey the views of users to policy makers. Moreover, her approach was one that stimulated other users to organise their own pressure groups.

The late 1990s and early part of the 20th century has seen a decline in the political influence of social workers at both central and local government levels. There is no social work spokesperson of Barbara's standing. The British Association of Social Workers (BASW) cannot be said to shape legislation. Today's children's services are often in the hands of highly paid people who have lost contact with social work practice. Child abuse cases result in huge attacks on social workers by both politicians and the press – a blame that is not generally directed at other participants, such as the police and health officials. Few social workers become MPs, so all political parties are distant from social work. In his exhaustive and exhausting account of the rise and fall of New Labour during 1997-2010, Andrew Rawnsley makes no mention of social work. New Labour's leaders frequently entertained celebrities and financiers at dinners and at Chequers, but social work leaders were not included (Rawnsley, 2010). And the succeeding Coalition government is practising the same exclusion. It is hard to avoid the conclusion that top politicians have little respect for social workers and pay minimal attention to what they say.

During the 1980s and 1990s, successful social work innovations were in evidence. Family centres were initiated by voluntary bodies and then taken on board by local authority social services departments. Their activities were varied and included day care for pre-school children, drop-in facilities for local parents, individual counselling, group meetings for those with problems such as drug addiction, heavy drinking and marital disharmony, involvement of local fathers in sport with each other and play with their children, toy libraries, voluntary classes for parents finding it difficult to cope with their children, and youth clubs. Two factors most had in common were that they tended to be located in deprived areas, and they emphasised parental strengths rather than labelling them as 'problem families'. Most family centres were a success in that they prevented children from being received into care, they improved the quality of life for some families and they were well-regarded by the local community (Holman, 1988, chapters 4-6).

Community social work entailed social workers being located near to the families they wanted to help, and encouraging local residents to set up facilities that served the area. The social workers often became adept at helping families receive their full benefits from social security and other sources.

In all, about 30% of social services departments set up what were called patch teams. In Easterhouse, Glasgow, a team was set up in disused flats. They contained a washing machine and a public telephone that drew in people who had kept away from social workers. Research demonstrated that the teams were accessible to needy families and that they did stimulate local action. Social workers and users looked more positively on each other. Some critics had predicted that the social workers' broad sweep would result in them giving less attention to children likely to be abused by the parents. In fact, child abuse was reduced, partly because the social workers became involved with the families at an early stage (Hadley and McGrath, 1984).

Despite the success of these innovations and despite the welcome awarded them by social workers, they declined almost to the point of extinction by the early years of the 20th century. Social workers and BASW were powerless to keep them in operation. In Easterhouse, local patch teams were closed and the social workers withdrawn to a new, huge building that was further away from users and required negotiating a system of buzzers to get in.

I would say that Tom White has been a social work leader of Barbara Kahan's calibre. Raised in a coalmining village in South Wales, he became a practising social worker and later the successful director of Coventry Social Services Department. Like Barbara, he was also a social work leader who negotiated with politicians and whose view carried weight. After serving Coventry for 15 years, he moved to head up the national voluntary society, the National Children's Home. On retirement, he refused to take advantage of what he called 'the consultancy gravy train' and was elected a councillor in Coventry. He was dismayed at what had happened to his old department, and wrote of what he saw in 1996:

> The structure of community based, locally accessible services, which I had strived so hard to create, had been judged too expensive and all service provision was now provided from specialist teams based in the centre of the city.... Most depressing of all, service managers still in the department from my day, would slide up to me and whisper or telephone to say how dangerously thinly spread the resources were, particularly in the protection of vulnerable children, where they feared a scandal would break any day. (White, 2010, pp 271-2)

And not just in Coventry. All over Britain, to this very day, heads of services – with some honourable exceptions – have been gripped by theories of management rather than social work, while central government insists on enormous cuts. The values and views of social workers count for little. Indeed, they have had to face reductions in their own salaries along with increases in their own workload. A survey of social workers by *Community Care* in 2011 found that 'Cuts in wages and rising living costs have left four in five social workers struggling to pay the bills' (*Community Care*, 2011b). Over half said that their disposable income had fallen by over £200 in a year, and in order to survive, many had had to sell items such as electrical goods, furniture or cars. A number had even sold their houses. A quarter had taken second jobs with the result that they often felt drained and exhausted during their social work hours. They had protested to their employers and to politicians. Some had gone on strike, but with little effect. Yet, for all their setbacks, most social workers remain loyal to their occupation and to the people they serve.

It is easy to say that social work needs the likes of Barbara Kahan today. It is easy to call on the leaders of statutory social work agencies to be as outspoken as she was. Certainly, I would ask them to be publicly on the side of their staff instead of 'going soft' on criticising politicians because they consider it fruitless, perhaps because they hope to become consultants and the recipients of honours. All I can suggest is the following.

- Social work spokespeople should seek to act in unison with organisations that represent users. They should show respect for each other and deliver a united front to those in central and local government.
- Political parties should increase the number of MPs from a social work background. Lawyers, financiers, businesspeople, former political advisers, are all over-represented in the House of Commons. For a start, the issue of which occupations are over- or under-represented should be raised at the annual conference of the major parties.
- Each political party should have an advisory committee made up of both social work managers and those who still work in the front line. It should meet as regularly as other advisory committees.

These suggestions are for the immediate future. Although Barbara tended to use her influence for the present and near future, nonetheless, I feel she would have been sympathetic towards contemporary thinkers and practitioners who believe that more profound change is now necessary. Iain Ferguson is one. He argues – rightly in my view – that neoliberal governments and the elites who shape Britain have attempted to make all state services subservient to the interests of the market and private business. He states that 'in Britain, every aspect of social work has been profoundly affected by the imposition of a culture of managerialism and competition' (Ferguson, 2008, p 3). In short, capitalism must rule.

A number of social services have now been privatised. When Barbara Kahan was at her height was at the height of her influence, the residential care of deprived children was largely in the hands of local authorities and not-for-profit voluntary bodies. Today 75% are run by private companies. In 2012, attention was drawn to them following the revelation that large numbers of the children were being sexually exploited and often running away. Randeep Ramesh called it 'an export trade in vulnerable children', and stated 'This risk has been heightened because private industry has set up clusters of care homes for vulnerable young people to save costs in cheaper areas – such as in the deprived north-west or along the coast' (Ramesh, 2012). It was not suggested that the private homes were involved in the sexual abuse, but rather that their choice of location gave too much priority to cheap rents. Maximising profit is a major if not the major aim. Some groups of homes change hands as they are bought and sold between companies. Advanced Child Care Ltd reported a turnover of £15 million in 2010. One private home charged £378,000 for some children, a fee met by local authorities.

Iain Ferguson concludes that the neoliberal governments 'have created a much more unequal society in which the lives of millions (including millions of children) can still be blighted by poverty' (2008, p 3). He looks to 'the creation of a different form of social work, rooted in social justice and more able to address the poverty, inequality and oppression that continue to be the lot of a majority of service users in the twenty-first century' (2008, p 7). Ferguson and his colleagues believe that they have a responsibility not just to provide the best services they can, but also to promote changes in the values and practices of a society that will allow these services to serve the interests of users rather than those of private enterprise.

John Stroud

John Stroud's child care novels are still read and sold, albeit in second-hand bookshops. In 2008, when the University of Birmingham celebrated 100 years of training social workers, it was pointed out that one of its most famous graduates was John Stroud. He may be remembered, but his great success in books and radio programmes of what child care social work was really like has all but disappeared.

John Stroud probably increased the popularity of these social workers, but no more. Now, many politicians and much of the media frequently condemn and scorn them. They are criticised for the months they take to place a child for adoption. Then they are blamed if adopters later find the child beyond their capacities to cope. They are attacked if they fail to remove children from parents where they are neglected or abused. A few days later, critics say they removed the children too quickly. Little is said or written about the day-to-day dogged work the same social workers undertake, and the fact that they often improve the lives of children.

I have a confession to make. Years ago I wrote a child care novel. Like John Stroud's first book, it was based on my own experiences. Unlike John Stroud, I did not have the courage to publish it under my own name, and it came out as written by Bob Laken (1984). It told of a community social worker who lived in a tough area, who formed close relationships with needy people and who involved residents in community action.

The book won a few reviews and all but one were positive. The exception was from a cleric who called it 'Christian pornography'. My hopes were raised when the publishers telephoned to say that TV had expressed an interest in a series about the community social worker. It never happened. The book was soon forgotten and the publishers were not interested in a follow-up. All I can say is that Amazon has two copies at the price of one penny each.

Social workers do sometimes appear in television and radio plays and occasionally in soaps. They are presented as caring, but rarely as effective. Their ability to provide long-term and skilful support is rarely conveyed. By contrast, police officers, doctors, soldiers and fire service staff are given bigger parts and may even be presented as heroes. Literature that features social workers as central characters has appeared, but few, if any, have the public influence of a John Stroud novel.

One publication has impressed me, however. Alistair Findlay is both a social worker and a poet. He served in the front line of social work in Scotland and England for 36 years, and was simultaneously a trade union activist. Somehow he found the time to publish two books of poems. On retirement he wrote another entitled *Dancing with Big Eunice: Missives from the front line of a fractured society* (2010). Big Eunice was a client and the front line is the demeaning circumstances in which the clients live.

I chortled and almost wept as I went from one poem to another. One is called 'Poverty':

> Poverty has a smell, it's kind of dank
> and musty, like you find gathered underneath
> a leaky sink, in cramped airless, overheated
> rooms, bare floorboards, carpets strewn with
> debris, but no toys, clutter, the junk that no one
> bothers to remove for no one notices the stink,
> and crunching underfoot, or calls growling dogs
> to heel, Alsatians mainly, that do quite literally
> steal the food from out the mouths of babes,
> whose sticky fingers point and stare and clamber
> over strangers' knees and poke your hair like
> you are long-lost cousins, not social workers
> only there to inspect the premises, motivations,
> a new lodger, lying on a chair not yet wakened.

All child care social workers have been in such homes. They do not make Findlay sneer or despair. Rather, the circumstances make him understand. He admires the parents who cope in these conditions. He perceives how family members defend each other before the social worker even if they also argue with each other. He does not condemn.

What does make him groan is the arrival of yet more paper instructions on his desk, as shown in the sarcastic poem 'Child protection guidelines (the latest)':

Lift up the phone, when the caller says 'abuse',
panic, over-react, run out of the door shouting
hysterically, send two social workers, also out
the door shouting hysterically, alert the police,
the zone paediatrician, ambulance service, fire-
brigade, health visitor, general practitioner,
midwife, Barnardo's, Tesco's, Dyno-Rod,
Visa, chief social work officer, child protection
register clerkess, her pal, the emergency duty
team, drug team, resources, criminal justice,
the Reporter to the Children's Hearing, the reviewing officer, the
area liaison coordinator's assistant for updating
the Scottish Executive's ongoing review of the
21st century social work's back-covering interim
consultative report, but don't, repeat don't
notify the parents, or ask the children anything, unless,
of course, you are accompanied by a police officer.

It brings a smile because we have all received useless advice 'from above'. It also raises a serious question. When did 'those above' last come face-to-face with a client? Findlay does appreciate some top officials, however, and praises Fred Edwards, Director of Social Work for Strathclyde, who gave material support to the families of striking miners, much to the anger of former Prime Minister, Margaret Thatcher. In a cynical yet humorous poem he has a go at managers in the poem 'Snap-shot':

Heard it all now – just had an e-mail –
the Corporate Manager, an Accountant
who used to be in charge of houses,
has been told by the Chief Executive,
an Accountant who used to be in charge
of wheelie-bins – what colour would you
like, madam? – who has told the Chief
Social Work Officer, who is now an
Accountant in charge of us, to offer up
a few ideas for a photo-shoot, now,
what this means is some grinning
councillor standing besides a wheel-chair,
not, I imagine, some child being forensically
examined for rape, a disaffected yob, an

ingrate, a doubly incontinent brain-damaged
inebriate, least of all, a drug-addict in prison
for injuring their child, because, you see,
and I suppose this is just a guess, but there
are just some things the great British public
just doesn't want to know about, or look at –
whether you photograph them, or not.

Findlay grieves that the real work of social workers does not get through
to the public. No wonder the public show little understanding or sympathy,
as displayed in his poem 'The radio phone-in':

where were the social workers
where were the grandparents
where were the friends and neighbours
exterminate the drug addicts
sterilise the drug addicts
stop the methadone programmes
what about the alcoholics
what about the criminals
what about the government
and
the final caller
stuff the do-gooders.

If you go to a party where you are not known, people always ask what
your job is. Our daughter is a doctor and got fed up when, after revealing
she was a doctor, the person talking promptly explained his/her symptoms.
She became a consultant in sexual health and thereafter replied that she
was a doctor who specialised in VD – no more medical questions! It can be
the same for social workers who meet the kind of comments in the above
poem. I used to side-track by saying I was a community social worker and
the silence that followed allowed me to ask the questions. Findlay conveys
that social workers often feel they are under attack on social occasions. His
way of coping with it has been a good sense of humour. His poem called
'The client said' pokes fun at his clients, but not in a cruel way:

The client said he was unaware
children were in the room
when he started rubbing his genitals

against the TV screen
because Gordon Brown came on
and he hates him.
The client said she took the children
to a friend in the early evening
before she started drinking
then decided to dreep (to drop)
from her second floor window
onto the bushes in the front garden.
The client said she burned
her left leg by pouring diesel
over it and setting it alight
but the pain got too much
so she thought if she drank
the rest it might knock her out.

Like many social workers, Findlay also copes by laughing at himself. Here is the first verse of a poem called 'Mrs McRobie':

Caught side of Davie McRobie bunking of school
while sitting at the traffic lights,
Graham's Road, saw his beatific face go from
shock to delight when I,
his social worker, crunched into the tail lights of a
truck that had moved off
then stopped, saw the wee bastard tug his mate's
coat, then run like fuck!

I have read thousands of pages about social work, brilliant research by academics, helpful analysis by practitioners, endless proposals by cabinet ministers for administrative re-organisations, yet none give the feel of social work like Alistair Findlay's poems. He conveys its sweat, its smell, its reality. He understands both its trivia and its enormity. He perceives why clients do what they do and what drives social workers to continue in their hard and thankless jobs. Unfortunately, *Dancing with Big Eunice* was not issued by a large, national publisher and so did not reach a huge audience, unlike the novels of John Stroud.

Social workers should be the main characters in a television serial, those who come over as professionals with faults that are outweighed by their positive contribution to society. This would inform millions about the much misunderstood occupation of social workers. But in my view, nothing replaces literature. From John Stroud to Alistair Findlay, it has been shown that social work can be brilliantly conveyed in words. Prizes for novelists and other writers abound. If only some institution would launch a major award for social work literature.

Clare Winnicott

The biography of Clare Winnicott, published in 2004, stimulated discussion of her contribution to the work of her husband, the child psychiatrist, Donald Winnicott (Kanter, 2004). She was often in the shadow of this man who, during the Second World War, had become famous as a broadcaster. It is worth mentioning that her interest in and expertise at child care casework developed before she met him. After training on the mental health course at the London School of Economics and Political Science (LSE), she opted to work with evacuees who were deemed to require residential care in hostels rather than family care with foster parents. She combined both administrating hostels and also relating individually with the children. For a while after the war, she worked with foster children and those expected to be placed for adoption. Her skills were recognised when she was appointed to the LSE to lead a new course to train child care officers.

She insisted that one of the main roles of these officers was to relate personally with the children for whom they were responsible, mainly those who were in the care of local authority children's departments or who were at risk of coming into care. In the chapter [in the original book on Clare Winnicott, I outlined the main themes in the lectures I heard her deliver. Child care officers had to discover the past experiences of the children, particularly those leading them to be removed from their own families, in order to understand how they could help them: they had to be the reliable person in their lives, the one to whom the children could turn with confidence and trust. They had to be adept at communicating with children so as to help them understand and deal with the rejections, the pain, the traumas they had endured – and might still face if they were moved to different families or residential homes while in public care. Not least, they had to identify, deal with and develop what Clare called 'the live bit' which is in every child. She called this 'child care casework', although today it is more likely to be called counselling.

During the 1950s and 1960s, child care casework was widely practised by child care social workers, many of whom recognised Clare Winnicott as their teacher and mentor. When I started as a child care officer, the area children's officer told me that, although administration was important, my priority was to relate with the children. It is a tragedy that this approach has declined.

Interestingly, Clare foresaw the decline when children's departments and other welfare services were absorbed into the much bigger social services departments in the 1970s. She acknowledged that the reform would win greater resources for social work, but feared that the specialism of child care would be diluted. At the same time, the Association of Child Care Officers, with which she had a close identification, was absorbed into BASW. Writing of BASW, Joel Kanter stated, 'Although she bravely welcomed the new organization, she never became active in its activities, and the personal approach to child care work that she and Donald advocated never found expression in the larger group' (Kanter, 2004, p 46). He added that since then, 'Too often our child care and child welfare systems have focussed on administrative and legal procedures, and the personal experience of child care is lost' (Kanter, 2004, p xi). This may be true, but it would be an exaggeration to say that child care casework has disappeared completely. The name 'child care officers' was replaced by the more embracing 'social workers', but some did still manage to give time to individual children, their parents and their carers, some did strive to continue their specialism and, in time, were called 'child care social workers'. Certainly, some social work courses still taught it and Clare herself delivered child care lectures on the social work course at LSE.

But other forces were also at work. The demands on social workers changed significantly due to the dominance given to child abuse by the media in the 1980s and onwards, due to the arrival of computers on social workers' desks in the 1990s and due to the cuts imposed on state agencies from 2010 following the election of the Coalition government. Official reports that blamed social work agencies for child deaths at the hands of their carers filled the front pages. Social work managers ordered their staff to see that all the right checks were being made on families and that reports and assessments and meetings were up to date. Administration rather than child care contact became the focus. At the conference to celebrate 100 years of social work training at the University of Birmingham, Professor of Social Work, Ann Davis, complained that social workers were very different from those in the old children's departments. She was reported as talking of 'Social workers sitting in front of screens for much of the day, often separated from the public at large by bars and security systems. The time spent writing reports now far exceeds time spent with clients' (Arnot, 2009). Her complaint was confirmed by a study reported by Anna Gupta that stated that social workers 'spend only a quarter of their time in direct contact with clients' (Gupta, 2010).

Time available for clients (or users) has become even more pressed as the Coalition government has imposed cuts on local authorities that has reduced the number of social workers. Children's services, often faced with growing demand for their under-manned services, have had to hire social workers from private agencies to cope. Paradoxically this is proving very expensive. No doubt some of these social workers are able and have turned to the private bodies because they cannot obtain permanent work with statutory services. But they do bring two disadvantages, as found by a study conducted by social work managers in the West Midlands. First, they tend not to stay long and so cannot provide the long-term attention required by some clients. Second, they sometimes lack the skills required for complex families (*Community Care*, October, 2011a).

I know many social workers, and believe that most regret the decline in child care casework. They see such work as valuable in helping clients who, whatever their financial circumstances, have deep-rooted problems which require skilled intervention on a one-to-one basis. Similarly with clients struggling with lesser emotional problems that affect the care of their children. They don't need threats or social workers acting as social police officers but professional friendships that set boundaries within a framework of encouragement. These social workers do not see child care casework or counselling as a means of diverting attention from the poverty that can undermine the capacity of parents to care fully for their children. Within positive relationships, they want to help them obtain their full benefits, prevent them from being evicted and ensure that they have access to quality day care. Overall, they regard relationships, often long-term, as a means by which clients can regain self-belief in themselves, despite the continual condemnation from politicians and the press, and in so doing, gain the confidence to relate with others in satisfactory ways.

How can child care casework be revived and shaped to help both those with problems which stem from rejection, separation and removal and also those whose despair, depression and humiliation is imposed by an unjust and unequal society? I can't pretend to have the answers, but a major step would be for politicians not to look on social workers as easy targets on which to direct blame when tragedies occur. Instead they should respect them as staff who often possess special skills that can be of huge benefit to vulnerable people. But this requires different conditions of work in which they have the time and backing to draw close to those in need. Power holders would do well to study the life of Clare Winnicott.

Peter Townsend

When Peter Townsend died on 7 June 2009, many glowing obituaries appeared in the press. And none was more moving than that issued by UNICEF, as follows, 'Peter Townsend will be missed by UNICEF, but even more by the millions of poor children around the world, who never heard his voice, but whom he never forgot in his research or in his advocacy nor most importantly, in his heart' (UNICEF, 2009).

Peter's friends organised a publication in his honour. Entitled *The Peter Townsend reader*, it contains selections from his writings introduced by academic experts. The range covers sociology and social policy, the welfare state and international welfare, poverty, inequality and social exclusion, health inequalities, older people, disability, and social justice and human rights (Walker et al, 2010). I want to highlight one of his shorter and less well-known articles that appeared in the collection. It is called 'The pursuit of equality' and was initially published in *Poverty*, CPAG's journal, in 1983. In it he dwells on two factors that he identified as of outstanding importance, and more recent studies now uphold his judgement.

Peter was always aware of inequality, the huge social and material differences between different sections of society. Sometimes he complained about 'the truce' over inequality in that all political parties largely ignored it. While he did not ignore the matter, he gave much more attention to poverty that he defined, studied and measured and, above all, which he campaigned to reduce and abolish. And with some success, because he succeeded in placing it on the public agenda. Indeed, a number of Conservative MPs gave their support to CPAG. But there was no Inequality Action Group.

He was, of course, the leading exponent of health inequalities, and established that among the many disadvantages suffered by poor people was their greater likelihood of suffering ill health. He saw these inequalities, as well as poverty, as something that sprang from inequality in general. In the 1980s, he placed much of his focus on inequality.

In 1983, he wrote a short article (re-published in *The Peter Townsend reader*). It was called 'The pursuit of equality' and appeared first in *Poverty*. It drew together his thinking of inequality that he was to enlarge in succeeding years.

In the article, Peter made clear the evil nature of inequality, and wrote eloquently 'about thoroughly unjust, undeserved and unnecessary exploitation and misery, on the one hand, and thoroughly unjust, undeserved and unnecessary assertion of power and wealth on the other' (quoted in Walker et al, 2010, p 295). He continued that greater equality was achievable, and explained, 'that the wealthiest 20 per cent of the population would only need to lose about a fifth of their present disposable income to finance a doubling of the incomes of the poorest 20 per cent' (quoted in Walker et al, 2010, p 299). Following this article, he did indeed pursue greater equality in his lectures and writings. He certainly succeeded in drawing greater attention to the existence of and the harm done by inequality, and asserted that the more equal society was a good society. However, his opponents usually retorted that those gaining more wealth actually benefited society by increasing total wealth, some of which, over time, filtered through to the poor.

In 2009, the very year in which Peter Townsend died, an outstanding book appeared that confirmed how right Peter had been to identify equality as the objective to be pursued. Richard Wilkinson and Kate Pickett examined over 200 reputable studies and compared unequal countries such as the US and Britain, where the top 20 per cent earned 7-9 per cent more than the lowest 20 per cent, with more equal countries such as Sweden, Finland and Norway, where the top 20 per cent earned only two to three times as much. Allen Lane published their findings in *The spirit level: Why more equal societies almost always do better.* The unequal countries scored higher on almost all social problems, physical and mental ill health, violence, teenage pregnancies, unemployment, child abuse, desertion by fathers, imprisonment and so on. Significantly, the higher scores applied to all classes. The authors stated, 'The truth is that the vast majority of the population is harmed by greater inequality' (Wilkinson and Pickett, 2009, back cover). Likewise, in more equal societies, those at the bottom had far fewer social disadvantages which, no doubt, contributed to the finding that, overall, these countries were far more contented. Peter Townsend's opponents were wrong – wealth at the top does not filter down in any marked way. The study vindicated his claim that greater equality should be pursued, both to give justice to those at the bottom and also for the good of every citizen.

His article 'The pursuit of equality' contained another important claim, namely, that inequality was not merely the refusal of the greedy rich to share with the needy poor, but was imbedded in the values and practices that dominated society. He identified the 'new individualism' of the Institute of Economic Affairs that influenced many politicians and economists. According to this, individuals should be free to accumulate money and power and the poor were to blame for their poverty. The economy this created led to more prosperity, more jobs, more stability – a view forwarded later not just by Conservatives but also by senior New Labour politicians. Peter argued that this view ignored the fact that the circumstances into which a person was born was the main determinant. Further, those with access to money and power were equipped to reinforce and maintain these inequalities. He stated:

> This line of analysis has a number of consequences. It means that the poverty and deprivation experienced by large sections of the population are not simply experiences which have arisen by chance or by misfortune and which only have to be publicised to ensure that countervailing action will be compelled by a sympathetic and receptive public opinion aided and abetted by liberal philosophers and politicians. They are experiences which flow directly and indirectly from the operations of industry, the banking system, the wage system and the property system generally, are condoned by the media and can be met only by action to reorganise such institutions. The argument has to be shifted from redistribution to production and distribution. A shift also has to be made from individualistic to social values. (quoted in Walker et al, 2010, pp 297-8)

In short, Peter Townsend was arguing that the contribution of charities such as CPAG was useful, but not sufficient. A more equal Britain required change to its economic and political system. Although the change did not come in his lifetime, some analytical challenges to the system have recently emerged. Peter would have been pleased to see a powerful one in the pages of *Poverty*.

Stewart Lansley, appropriately a visiting fellow at the Townsend Centre for International Poverty Research at the University of Bristol, wrote a piece which attacked the theory that lower taxes for those at the top increase wealth and bring economic stability, while everyone benefits financially. In other words, inequality is a virtue. Examining economic developments since 1945, Lansley demonstrates that these conditions have the outcome that 'The income gap has surged but without the promised pay-off of wider economic progress.... Not only has inequality failed to deliver faster growth, there is growing evidence that it is also associated with greater instability and played a critical role in both the 2008 Crash and the persistence of the current slump' (Lansley, 2012). The reasons for these outcomes were that the fall in incomes of those at the bottom reduced their purchasing power that had helped the economy grow. The swollen corporate and personal wealth, 'Instead of boosting investment ... led to a giant mountain of footloose global capital'. Not least, the concentration of wealth also led to a concentration of power akin to Victorian times in which 'economic decision making is heavily concentrated in the hands of a tiny minority' (Lansley, 2012). By contrast, 'the most prolonged period of economic success and stability – from 1950 to the early 1970s – was one in which inequality fell and the proceeds of growth were evenly shared between wages and profits and across earnings groups' (Lansley, 2012).

Lansley concludes that 'The pursuit of more equal societies needs to be elevated to a primary goal of domestic and global economic policy' (Lansley, 2012). His economic analysis lends support to the social analysis of Peter Townsend. Social justice for the poor, the unequal, the oppressed, cannot come just from better management and agency reforms. In the long run, it will require the spread of democracy so that political decision making is not largely restricted to political and financial elites. It will require the replacement of the dominance of personal greed by a respect for all people and the promotion of the common good. In short, the kind of society in which Peter Townsend believed.

Over a decade since the first issue of this book, I have selected six contemporary issues about which the six child care champions still have relevance. The issues vary enormously:

- Greater respect for and better understanding of the parents of poor children (Eleanor Rathbone) is not of interest to cabinet ministers, but would do much to improve their confidence.
- Better play facilities for children (Marjorie Allen) is unlikely to hit the headlines, but could give enormous enjoyment to them.
- Child care novels and poems (John Stroud) but they offer insights into the lives of families in need of help.
- Child care casework will not get a mention in the Common, but is the neglected means of communicating with those who are often at a distance from society (Clare Winnicott).
- More praise and influence for social workers (Barbara Kahan) is hardly the subject of editorial leaders, but they are essential to the well-being of many vulnerable children.
- A more equal society (Peter Townsend) seems almost too big for a book about children's champions, but such a society means the decrease of many of the social problems that blight countless lives.

So these champions still have something to offer.

Bob Holman

When this book was first published in 2001, my wife, Annette, and I were still living in Easterhouse, Glasgow, where I was a volunteer and committee member of the locally run project, Family Action in Rogerfield and Easterhouse (FARE) that was located in six flats. In 2004 we moved across

Glasgow to look after our grandchildren, Lucas and Nathan, while both their parents worked. I continued as a volunteer at FARE and we both remained members of Easterhouse Baptist Church.

We were still in Easterhouse when, in 2002, FARE was asked if the leader of the Conservative Party, Iain Duncan Smith, could visit it. He was trying to show that Conservatives could be compassionate and was also going to other voluntary agencies. FARE's committee was ready to welcome and inform any politician, but in subsequent years, some members of the Labour Party levelled criticism at FARE for its connection with Duncan Smith.

On arrival he was friendly and ready to learn. And learn he did. Coming from a socially sheltered background of an affluent family, boarding school and Sandhurst, he was deeply moved at the reality of poverty. He realised that some people were living on very low incomes in damp flats. In a street where children played, he spotted a needle, thrown away by a drug user. At FARE, he was impressed at the skills and motivations of residents who helped to run the project, particularly lone parents and unemployed people. He remarked that these were the very people that Maggie (Thatcher) had criticised. After leaving, he announced his two intentions. One was to tackle poverty. He stated, 'When I visited Glasgow, I saw the poverty, the crime, the drug abuse.... I felt I had to do something. I came away a changed man' (*Community Care*, 2004). The other was that locally run community groups would receive funding from central government, so that if they raised £1,000 locally, central funds would add £2,000.

After losing the leadership of his party in 2003, he could have opted for the easy money of private consultancies and directorships. Instead he founded The Centre for Social Justice. There I met one of its part-time staff, Andy Stranack, who was standing as a Conservative candidate in the next election. He wanted to put his Christian principles into practice and, despite having difficulties in walking due to childhood cerebral palsy, he had left a well-paid job to live in a deprived area on a low income.

Meanwhile, his radicalism seemed to increase. In 2005, he agreed to speak at a fringe meeting of the Labour Party Conference in Manchester. He criticised the New Labour government for allowing inequality to widen. Then he declared it needed a more realistic measure of poverty, saying, 'We should understand that poverty is not just about a lack of basics but a lack of sufficient resources to live in the community' (Christian Socialist Movement, 2005).

When the Conservatives did come to power, Iain Duncan Smith was appointed Minister for Work and Pensions, and soon announced plans for a universal credit scheme that would both simplify the complex welfare system and tackle poverty. As I explained in the press, he was soon blaming the poor for their own poverty and punishing them by imposing drastic cuts (Holman, 2012a). There was no new definition of poverty while the rich got richer and the poor got poorer. I argued that the enormous cuts in the welfare budget imposed by George Osborne, Chancellor of the Exchequer, had made it impossible for Duncan Smith to achieve his aims. I called on him to resign and become an independent campaigner against poverty.

In late 2012, the Christian journal *Third Way* published an interview with Duncan Smith, in which he acknowledged that in his post he had found it hard to make compromises, saying, 'They are difficult these compromises. Particularly in a time of austerity, it's really hard to make these changes because you are also being asked to make savings.' The interviewer, Huw Spanner, then asked about the criticisms I had made about him. He replied graciously, 'I think it is quite legitimate for someone like Bob to tell me that I've done something wrong – and it does make me pause for thought. I sit and reflect, maybe he is right, maybe I could have done more to stop something and perhaps I got engaged in the ghastly game of government too much.' When Huw Spanner asked about my suggestion that he resign and be a public campaigner for social justice, he said, 'I know. I would love to do that and who knows that at some point I won't?' (Spanner, 2012).

I now turn from high government to life on a housing scheme. During the years from 2001, FARE gradually expanded its outreach. The gangs in Easterhouse had long been a cause for public concern. Indeed, the large space to the back of FARE's building was known as 'the killing fields' as fights sometimes took place there. The committee agreed with its leader, Rosemary Dickson, on what was called a territorial strategy. Initially, staff – some of whom had been gang members – went into schools to discuss with pupils the reasons why gangs functioned, why they were attractive and why they were dangerous. Next, clubs and sporting activities were promoted in each of the neighbourhoods where gangs were prominent. Then came the hardest part, joint activities. The gangs played each other at football, went on outings and did the Duke of Edinburgh's award together, visiting each other's clubs. There were scary times, but overall it worked. After three years, Strathclyde police announced a decrease of 58.9% in 'targeted crime, vandalism and youth disorder'. Glasgow City Council funded much of the work.

Another initiative to bring younger children together came in an annual Olympic Games held indoors at the Kelvin Hall sports centre and funded by the local housing association. Schools in Greater Easterhouse entered teams – there were 19 at the last event in 2012. Six weeks before it started,

FARE's staff went into the schools to enthuse and train the children. They have been a great success with hundreds of children (and parents) attending, with friendly rivalry but no trouble. Medals are presented to all the winners. I was asked to award a cup to the best school. As I had always been hopeless at athletics, I called it the Cup for Sporting Spirit. The children themselves vote for the winner but cannot vote for their own school. I was pleased when a school that did not win one race won the trophy in 2012.

FARE's building became too small, however, and it was likely that the tenement blocks in the street would be demolished. The committee made the brave decision to go for a new building. This was encouraged by a report from New Philanthropy Capital that gave FARE its seal of approval, explaining to potential donors that FARE gave a high quality service to young people, had developed a grassroots approach and had improved the well-being of the area.

The raising of £1.6 million owed much to staff members, with Graham Allison working full time on it. Iain Montague, born and bred just a few yards from the new site, had been treasurer since FARE started, and contacted and impressed a number of charitable grant givers. Local Member of the Scottish Parliament (and later the MP) Margaret Curran, John Mason, also an MSP and member of Easterhouse Baptist Church, and local councillors gave their backing. Another source of help was TV personality, Duncan Bannatyne, who himself had been brought up in working-class Glasgow and could communicate with local young people. He lent FARE one of his managers who was adept at negotiating with the builders and local suppliers, and must have saved FARE thousands of pounds.

The new building, spacious and well equipped, was opened in November 2010. It stands next to Lochfield Housing Association that gave its support. It is near the old building but located on a road that divides two territories, and young people from both neighbourhoods have become part of FARE. Club attendances are much higher than before – in 2010-11 there were 57,000 attendances in all. In addition, staff help at 10 outreach clubs. A new development has been to third and fourth year pupils in secondary schools to enhance employability prospects by the time they leave school. Of 180 young people, 31 have gained jobs, 51 have gone into further education and 80 into further training.

With more facilities, FARE has expanded its work with adults, to include voluntary parenting classes, IT training, parent and toddler groups, carpet bowls, family bike rides, walking groups for the over-60s, Zumba dancing and an enthusiastic knitting group.

Elderly people (and needy families) received 600 parcels at Christmas. Financed by the Charity Advisory Trust, the goods are packed with the help of school children and then delivered by both an adult and a child. The parcels contain mostly food. One elderly man wept as he said, "With a bit less to spend on food, I can keep the heating on longer." Loss of jobs, frozen benefits and higher food prices have hit Easterhouse residents. FARE has re-introduced the sale of cheap nappies, and sometimes a parent buys one nappy. This very morning, I was arranging our annual under-canvas camp and some parents are struggling to pay the fee. Yet just as more people are turning to FARE, so its grants have been cut. Three members of staff were to be made redundant. Other workers took an 8 per cent cut in their own modest salaries so that they could be retained. One excellent youth worker who left for another post could not be replaced. Iain Duncan Smith appears to have forgotten about his pledge to ensure that groups such as FARE should receive extra funding from central government.

FARE was not in a neighbourhood that housed asylum seekers. When we moved across Glasgow, Annette and I found ourselves close to a tower block that accommodated a number of asylum seekers. They were often in poor conditions and with little money because they were not allowed to work. We met several in the drop-in centre of the local church. One family had fled their country after their business had been ransacked by the army and a relative had been shot and killed. We became friends, went for tea in their flat where the wife insisted on cooking something, and accompanied them to their mosque. They were gentle, polite, intelligent people with delightful children. One day they skipped into the centre and announced that – after five years – they had been granted asylum. We all rose to our feet, clapped, cheered and wept. They were a part of us. Not long after, I stood at the bottom of the tower block while aggressive immigration officials forced their way into a 20th floor flat where a wife collapsed in fright and was rushed to hospital. The children were removed. The husband clung to the balcony until finally taken out. Soon after, against their will, they were all on a plane back to their war-torn home country.

I asked Iain Duncan Smith to set up a working group under the auspices of his Centre for Social Justice. This was before he was in government and I must praise him for responding quickly. Its members were not politicians but experts on asylum issues, staff of agencies that helped asylum seekers, an asylum seeker and myself as vice-chair. Its report, *Asylum matters*, found that many applicants for asylum received unsympathetic treatment from some officials. In Glasgow, I met a number of female asylum seekers who had been sexually abused but did not feel they could discuss it with their interviewers. In 2004, only 3% obtained permission to stay at their initial application, but 30% who went to appeal before judges had the decision reversed.

Many asylum seekers whose applications were rejected refused to go home. They disappeared underground in order to avoid been forced to leave, and survived on meagre casual earnings or lived rough. I met two young men from Zimbabwe sleeping on benches in Glasgow. When I asked why they did not go back they replied, "This is better than torture." I visited several voluntary bodies – often churches – that provided food, clothes and shelter from their limited funds. In Newcastle, I met a woman who had been imprisoned for her political activities, who had escaped and had found her way to Britain where her application to stay was turned down. She wept as she told me that, at times, she had resorted to prostitution in order to buy food.

I also went to the Boaz Trust in Manchester where, unusually, it provides accommodation, although it is never enough. One woman told me that she had had to flee so quickly that her children got left behind. She could rarely afford to telephone or write to them. To re-join them would mean torture and worse. The pain was etched in her face.

The New Labour and Conservative governments have displayed insufficient concern for asylum seekers. A Mori poll in 2007 discovered that the average person believes that Britain receives 23% of the world's asylum seekers. The politicians rarely point out that the real figure is less than 2%. They are hostile to asylum seekers because it is a vote winner.

The main recommendations of the Working Group – which were approved by Iain Duncan Smith – were three-fold. First, that the initial decision making for asylum application should be undertaken not by immigration officials but by an independent body of trained, lay judges. Second, at hearings, all applicants should be properly represented. And third, those rejected should be offered help from skilled volunteers to advise them whether and how to appeal or, if they wished, how best to return to their own country (The Centre for Social Justice, 2008).

I add two more recommendations. That those who are in the midst of making applications be allowed to work. Many are highly skilled, often professional people, and their salaries would ease their poverty and mean that public money would not be required for their support. Voluntary bodies, that help rejected applicants, should receive statutory grants so that they can avoid destitution. No major political party has shown interest in these recommendations. I put them forward here as proposals that would give dignified help to one of the most misunderstood and oppressed minorities in Britain.

In 2009, I went through various medical tests. Then I was suddenly called to hospital. The consultant kindly but firmly said, "I'm sorry Mr Holman, the biopsy shows you have cancer." It was Hodgkin's Lymphoma, cancer of the lymph glands, that had spread to other organs. Soon I was undergoing six months' chemotherapy. The side effects included sickness, tiredness, my finger nails dropping off and losing my hair. Our youngest grandson, Nathan, nicknamed me "Baldy Bob".

I was not afraid of death but, at times, I experienced great sadness at what I might lose. We live in a small, ex-council house that might not be sought after for its beauty. Yet from the bedroom window I could see blossom in the spring and russet leaves in the autumn on a neighbour's tree. It had long given me a sense of wonder that I wanted to retain. Above all, I could not bear the thought of being parted from my family.

Another drawback was that, as my immunity to infections was low, I had to avoid crowds and public transport. I could not take my grandson Lucas on a promised trip to see my West Ham United lose again. I was allowed to go to church but only once a fortnight, I had to sit at the back, wear gloves, and shun any cuddles or kisses – which was difficult in our loving fellowship.

There was compensation, however. I had never had so many visitors. Two young men, hearing I was ill, came to see me. Both had attended the youth clubs that I had helped to run in Easterhouse. One was employed as a residential social worker. The other was in the army and expecting to be posted overseas (he later went to Afghanistan). Both indicated that their years in the clubs had diverted them from gangs and trouble. In Easterhouse, I had often been the visitor. Now I was the visited, and it made me feel valued as an individual, yet also a member of like-minded people. And above all, I felt even closer to my wife, Annette, who, as a former medical social worker, understood more about illness than me. She became my nurse, always accompanying me on consultations, making sure I rested, ensuring that I took the numerous pills, and above all, talking with me, as no one else could, about the deep things of life and thereafter. Our friends nicknamed her 'matron'. I hated cancer yet, strangely, it was an experience that deepened my understanding of myself and made me aware how much others loved me.

I went to our GP and hospital for numerous consultations, tests, minor operations and chemotherapy, and the care I received was beyond measure. The cancer consultant was considerate, explained carefully what was happening, offered hope, yet never promised that recovery was certain. When I started to improve I told her that, as always, I would be going with Easterhouse youngsters on its annual under-canvas camp. She warned me that recovery would take longer than I realised, but for once she was wrong. I got there. I was an in-patient for a couple of periods and I especially appreciated an assistant who both swept the ward and, late at night, made tea and toast for us all. I can remember the birth of the NHS in 1948 and how my parents – who were not political people – rejoiced that they would then receive a free and high standard service. I now want to do all I can to halt the creeping privatisation of the NHS.

One other compensation of the illness was that, often confined to home, I had more time to write. I was able to complete a book on Keir Hardie, probably Scotland's greatest political figure. Born in dire poverty in 1856, he had virtually no school education. A coalminer, he was sacked for his trade union activities. Soon after, he became a Christian and then a socialist. In 1892, he stood as a parliamentary candidate in West Ham South and won a surprising and sensational victory. He built up the Labour Party and became its first leader in the Commons.

What impressed me about Hardie was not just his great political achievements; it was his insistence on putting principles into practice in the way he lived. He never pursued money or honours. When the Liberal Party offered him a safe seat and a large salary, at a time when MPs were not paid, he turned it down. For much of their lives, he and his loyal wife, Lillie, survived on his meagre earnings from articles and talks. They grew their own vegetables and Hardie never travelled anything but third class. He declined invitations to eat with the wealthy or to join the clubs of the powerful, and always stayed close to the people he served. He died in 1915. No Conservative or Liberal MPs attended his funeral in Glasgow but hundreds of working-class men and women marched behind him on his last journey. At a memorial service, Mary Macarthur, by then a well-known trade union leader, rose to speak. She recalled how, when the leader of a struggling union of telephone girls, she sought out Hardie in the Commons. She said, 'As he was speaking to me, one of the great and mighty ones came up and began praising something he had done. Hardie looked at him stiffly and coldly and said, "I am engaged just now"' (quoted in Holman, 2010). Although tired, he left to meet the telephone girls. Typically, he was offended by the mighty and welcoming to the needy.

I had told Annette that Hardie was my last book, but when Lion Hudson asked me to write a life of Woodbine Willie, I could not refuse because I had been inspired by him since reading his poems – or rhymes – as a teenager. Born in 1883, Geoffrey Studdert Kennedy, to use his proper name, served as a priest, with his wife Emily, in a poor parish in Worcester. With the outbreak of the First World War, he enlisted as a chaplain, convinced that Britain was right to fight. He was able to communicate with ordinary soldiers to whom he distributed cigarettes on their way to battle – hence the nickname Woodbine Willie. He also accompanied them to the front line and won the military cross. But the wholesale and needless slaughter changed him.

After the war, he resumed as a parish priest. He disliked the way in which the affluent distanced themselves from the poor. He spent much of his time 'in the houses squashed into back-to-back terraces. Some evenings he would laugh and sing in the local pub before going to sit with the poor sick and dying in their cold homes' (Holman, 2013). His fame as Woodbine Willie won him many invitations to speak. By this time he was anti-war and angry that, despite government promises to end poverty, it continued. The following statements are typical, 'I believe that hungry children and child waste make God Almighty mad'; 'We (the church) do not recognise class distinctions in any form'; and 'If God wills war then am morally mad and I don't know God from evil' (quoted in Holman, 2012b). Before long he was a full-time national speaker who drew enormous crowds and publicity. He also wrote best-selling books and volumes of rhymes that explained Christianity in straightforward language. Worn out, he died in 1929, at the age of 45.

Studdert Kennedy had little faith in political parties. He believed that the lead had to come from the church that could change people morally, so that concern for others, particularly the poor, became a common practice. He thus had a different approach from Keir Hardie, but they had one thing in common. He lived out his beliefs. In an age when most bishops were drawn from those who went to public schools and Oxbridge, his own humble background meant he had little chance of ecclesiastical promotion. He was glad because he believed that Christians – like Christ – should be close to the poor. He never took more than a modest salary. He did receive large royalties for his books and, typically, he gave it all away, mainly to charities. While a priest in Worcester, he and Emily took their bed to a woman who was dying on the floor of her home. If he saw a person without shoes or clothes, he took off his own. When he died, he left very little.

The poor and unemployed flocked to the funerals of Keir Hardie and Studdert Kennedy. They were loved. My studies of them found that, as well as preaching to thousands, they had a great influence over numerous individuals who were drawn by the way they lived.

This epilogue has drawn on the children's champions to propose social reforms large and small. Readers who are political and social activists will continue to agitate, argue, campaign for these changes, but the chances of creating a much more equal society appear small. Nobel prize winner, Joseph Stiglitz, in his brilliant *The price of inequality: The avoidable causes and hidden costs of inequality*, shows how neoliberal ideologies have a complete grasp on much of Western society so that inequality is increasing (Stiglitz, 2012). For me, the most depressing part is how the Labour Party has contributed to this. I see some former socialists who, on becoming MPs, have been seduced by the higher circles in which they move and who have succumbed to the lust for power and money and have ended up with their honours, their titles, their consultancies, their expensive homes – and their distance from the poor. They are a now part of the problem. They may hold the power but there is one thing they cannot stop us doing, namely, following the example of Keir Hardie and Studdert Kennedy.

We can choose more modest lifestyles, but I am not proposing that, if in top jobs, we should abandon them. Rather, it is about being satisfied with a portion of our income and giving any residue to those in need or to the agencies that support them. We can reduce spending on large cars, wall-to-wall televisions, electronic gadgets, costly holidays, the latest fashion in clothes and classy restaurants and hotels. This does not entail living like a monk or nun. Rather, it means giving less priority to material possessions and more to the well-being of others.

We do not have to put our savings in the financial institution where it gets the most interest regardless of its lack of ethics. While the High Street banks tend to stimulate greed and inequality, the Co-operative Bank, which has grown significantly of late, did not make the risky loans that contributed to the credit crisis, did not shed thousands of jobs, and did not pay huge bonuses to its top managers and directors. Its members have a say in its ethical policies, one of which is to have no dealings with companies engaged in the arms trade. I joined it over 25 years ago when it was the only bank that could convince me that it played no part at all in reinforcing apartheid in South Africa. There are other banks, although small in number, based on similar principles, as well as several mutual building societies. Credit unions are strong on local involvement and make low interest loans. As a member of one in Easterhouse, I know that it helps some residents who might otherwise fall into the hands of legal or illegal loan sharks.

We can also choose to do at least some of our shopping in Co-operative food shops. They are responsible to members and not shareholders and, unlike the huge private supermarkets, do not use profits to enrich directors and top staff. Every day I go to a Co-op shop where I have got to know the staff. Like other Co-op shops it gives prominence to fair trade goods and has strong trading links with Malawi. It is a part of the community and supports local charities. I also insure with the Co-op, use its pharmacy and will be buried by it – with my wife giving the divi to charity. It is not well known that the Co-operative group is one of the largest farm owners in Britain that cares for its environment, and with every farm having beehives with Co-op money also funding research to understand why so many bees are dying. Not least, the Co-operative Party is backing and proposing a range of different kinds of cooperatives, ranging from football clubs to the railways.

Many of us have some choice as to where we live. I am not suggesting that we should all move to very deprived areas, but some might consider homes in cheaper, less fashionable places. Yes, it would be a financial sacrifice in that such homes do not increase in value so quickly. The social gain is that it puts us closer to people on low incomes. It would promote contact with more people who are helped (or not) by social security and social services. We could become part of their community, send our children to their schools and support local shops. Not least, we could campaign and act with, not just for, residents in order to improve the neighbourhood.

These practices are important. They challenge the evils of greed and selfishness. They are a lifestyle that expresses the wish for an end to poverty and a socially divided society. They display a commitment to commercial and social services that serve and respect people rather than using and regarding them as no more than economic units. If the participants multiply in number, they might even exert pressure on politicians to build the kind of society that reflects the values of the champions.

References

Arnot, C. (2009) 'Ann Davis, professor of social work', *Guardian Society*, 28 January.

Butterworth, E. and Holman, R. (1975) *Social welfare in modern Britain*, Glasgow: Fontana/Collins.

Campbell, D. and Butler, P. (2012) 'Half of all teachers say they bring in food for poor pupils', *The Guardian*, 20 June.

Centre for Social Justice, The (2008) *Asylum matters*, London: The Centre for Social Justice, chapter seven.

Child Poverty Action Group, (2011) Letter to members, 25 November.

Christian Socialist Movement (2005) *Can the Tories do social justice?*, Christian Socialist Movement.

Community Care (2004) 'Road to Damascus', 22-28 July.

Community Care (2011a) 'Over-paid and under-skilled: report slams agency children's social workers', 7 October.

Community Care (2011b) 'A quarter of social workers have second jobs', 13 October.

CPAG (Child Poverty Action Group) (2011) Letter to members, 25 November.

Findlay, A. (2010) *Dancing with Big Eunice: Missives from the front line of a fractured society*, Edinburgh: Luath Press.

Ferguson, I. (2008) *Reclaiming social work*, London: Sage Publications.

Guardian, The (2012) 'Duncan Smith wants City to help in tackling causes of social breakdown', 13 March.

Gupta, A. (2010) 'Root and branch review of sector', *Community Care*, 22 April.

Hardy, R. (2005) 'Doing good and winning love: social work and fictional autobiographies by Charles Dickens and John Stroud', *British Journal of Social Work*, volume 35, issue 2, pp. 207-22.

Hadley, R. and McGrath, M. (1984) *When social services are local*, London: Allen & Unwin.

Hamilton, J. (2012) 'Trips cut as incomes squeezed', *The Guardian*, 5 March.

Hardy, R. (2005) 'Doing good and winning love: social work and fictional autobiographies by Charles Dickens and John Stroud', *British Journal of Social Work*, vol 35, issue 2, pp 207-22.

Herald, The (2012a) 'Playgrounds may get £1.5bn budget', 9 June.

Herald, The (2012b) 'Cameron in 2bn benefits cut warning', 25 June.

Holman, B. (1988) *Putting families first*, London: Macmillan Education.

Holman, B. (2010) *Keir Hardie: Labour's greatest hero?*, Oxford: Lion Hudson.

Holman, B. (2012a) 'Iain Duncan Smith should resign, says Bob Holman', *The Guardian*, 20 June.

Holman, B. (2013) *Woodbine Willie: An unsung hero of World War One*, Oxford: Lion Hudson.

Kahan, B. (1980) *Growing up in care*, Oxford: Blackwell.

Kanter, J. (ed) (2004) *Face to face with children: The life and work of Clare Winnicott*, London: Karnac.

Laken, B. (1984) *More than a friend*, Oxford: Lion.

Lansley, S. (2012) 'Inequality and instability', *Poverty*, issue 142, pp 10-13.

Observer, The (2012) 'We must not abandon the battle against child poverty', 10 June.

Philpot, T. (2000) 'Child care pioneer whose "Pindown" scandal report prompted residential care reform', *The Guardian*, 9 August.

Policy Press, ed, (2010) *The Peter Townsend Reader*, Bristol: The Policy Press.

Ramesh, R. (2012) 'Export trade in children to end', *The Guardian*, 3 June.

Rawnsley, A. (2010) *The end of the party: The rise and fall of New Labour*, London: Penguin Books.

Shildrick, T. (2012) 'Low pay, no pay churning', *Poverty*, issue 142, pp 4-9.

Spanner, H. (2012) 'Quiet resolve', *Third Way*, Autumn.

Stewart, H. (2011) 'Working for nothing', *The Observer*, 20 October.

Stiglitz, J. (2012) *The price of inequality: The avoidable causes and hidden costs of inequality*, London: Allen Lane.

UNICEF (2009) 'UNICEF mourns death of Peter Townsend', Statement, 15 June.

Walker, A., Gordon, D. and Levitas, R. (eds) (2010) *The Peter Townsend reader*, Bristol: The Policy Press.

White, T. (2010) *The surprise of my life*, Chipping Norton: Tom White.

Wilkinson, R. and Pickett, K. (2009) *The spirit level: Why more equal societies almost always do better*, London: Allen Lane.

Bibliography

Abel-Smith, B. and Townsend, P. (1965) *The poor and the poorest*, London: Bell.

Alberti, J. (1996) *Eleanor Rathbone*, London: Sage Publications.

Allen, M. (1945) *Whose children?*, London: The Favil Press.

Allen, M. (1953) *Adventure playgrounds*, London: National Playing Fields Association.

Allen, M. (1968) *Planning for play*, London: Thames and Hudson.

Allen, M. (1973) *Adventure playgrounds for handicapped children*, London: Handicapped Adventure Playground Association.

Allen, M. and Nicholson, M. (1975) *Memoirs of an uneducated Lady*, London: Thames and Hudson.

Attlee, C. (1954) *As it happened*, London: Heinemann.

Beveridge, W. (1942) *The report on social insurance and allied social services* (Beveridge Report), London: HMSO.

Birmingham Post, The (1970) 'Ennals in clash on poverty budget', 20 April.

Bowlby, J. (1953) *Child care and the growth of love*, Harmondsworth: Penguin Books.

Bowlby, J., Miller, E. and Winnicott, D. (1939) Letter in *British Medical Journal*, 16 December, reprinted in C. Winnicott, R. Shepherd and M. Davis (eds) (1984, reprinted 1997) *Deprivation and delinquency: D. W. Winnicott*, London: Routledge.

Bradshaw, J. (2000) 'Child poverty in comparative perspective', in D. Gordon and P. Townsend (eds) *Breadline Europe: The measurement of poverty*, Bristol: The Policy Press.

Brand, J. (1999) 'You can't measure our commitment', letter in *Community Care*, 9-15 December.

Bridge Child Care Development Service (1997) *Report of the Bridge Child Care Development Service on Ricky Neave*, Cambridge: Cambridgeshire Social Services Department.

Brill, K. (1991) 'The Curtis experiment', PhD thesis, Birmingham: Birmingham University.

Britton, C. (1st edn, 1949, 2nd edn, 1954) 'Child care', in C. Morris (ed) *Social case-work in Great Britain*, London: Faber and Faber.

Burt, C. (1925) *The young delinquent*, London: University of London Press.

Carey, J. (1950) *Charley is my darling*, London: Michael Joseph.

Cohen, B. and Rea Price, J. (1996) 'Introduction', in K. Tidsall (ed) *Child welfare*, Edinburgh: HMSO.

Coles, C. (1961) *Michael O'Leary*, London: Victory Press.

Cooper, J. (1984) 'Clare Winnicott: sustaining a generation of social workers', *Community Care*, 10-16 May.

CPAG (Child Poverty Action Group) (1965) *Family policy memorandum to the Prime Minister*, London: CPAG.

Davies, A. (1992) *To build a new Jerusalem: The labour movement from the 1880s to the 1990s*, London: Michael Joseph.

DHSS (Department of Health and Social Security) (1974a) *Report of the committee on one-parent families* (Finer Report), London: HMSO.

DHSS (1974b) *Report of the committee of inquiry into the care and supervision in relation to Maria Colwell*, London: HMSO.

DHSS (1980) *Inequalities in health: Report of a working group* (Black Report), London: DHSS.

DHSS and the Welsh Office (1977) *Working together for children and their families*, London: HMSO.

DoH (Department of Health) (1997) *People like us: The report of the review of the safeguards for children living away from home* (Utting Report), London: The Stationery Office.

DoH (1998a) *Independent inquiry into inequalities in health* (Acheson Report), London: DoH.

DoH (1998b) *The government's response to the children's safeguards review*, London: The Stationery Office.

Donnison, D. (1982) *The politics of poverty*, London: Martin Robertson.

Donnison, D. (2001) *Towards a more equal society*, Nottingham: Spokesman Books.

Field, F. (1982) *Poverty and politics*, London: Heinemann.

Field, F. (1996a) 'The whisper of greatness: Eleanor Rathbone 50 years on', Talk to the Holocaust Trust, 5 February.

Field, F. (1996b) 'A family legacy', *The Guardian*, 7 February.

Fox Harding, L. (1991) *Perspectives in child care policy*, Harlow: Longman.

Gibbons, J. with Thorpe, S. and Wilkinson, P. (1990) *Family support and prevention*, London: HMSO.

Goldstein, J., Freud, A. and Solnit, A. (1973) *Beyond the best interests of the child*, New York, NY: The Free Press.

Goldstein, J., Freud, A. and Solnit, A. (1979) *Before the best interests of the child*, New York, NY: The Free Press.

Gordon, D. and Townsend, P. (eds) (2000) *Breadline Europe: The measurement of poverty*, Bristol: The Policy Press.

Gordon, D., Pantazis, C. and Townsend, P. (2000) 'Absolute and overall poverty: a European history and proposal for measurement', in D. Gordon and P. Townsend (eds) *Breadline Europe: The measurement of poverty*, Bristol: The Policy Press.

Hague, W. (1999) Speech to *Community Care Live* Conference, 15 December.

Hartley, M. (1999) Letter in *Community Care*, 29 July-4 August.

Hendrick, H. (1993) *Child welfare in England 1872-1989*, London: Routledge and Kegan Paul.

Heywood, J. (1959) *Children in care*, London: Routledge and Kegan Paul.

Holman, B. (1973) *Trading in children: A study of private fostering*, London: Routledge and Kegan Paul.

Holman, B. (1975) 'The place of fostering in social work', *British Journal of Social Work*, vol 5, no 1, pp 3-29.

Holman, B. (1976) *Inequality in child care*, London: Child Poverty Action Group.

Holman, B. (1978) *Poverty: Explanations of social deprivation*, London: Martin Robertson.

Holman, B. (1981) *Kids at the door*, Oxford: Blackwell.

Holman, B. (1988) *Putting families first: Prevention and child care*, Basingstoke: Macmillan Education.

Holman, B. (1990) *Good old George: The life of George Lansbury*, Oxford: Lion Publishing.

Holman, B. (1993) *A New Deal for social welfare*, Oxford: Lion Publishing.

Holman, B. (1995) *The evacuation: A very British revolution*, Oxford: Lion Publishing.

Holman, B. (1996) *The corporate parent. Manchester Children's Department 1948-1971*, London: National Institute for Social Work.

Holman, B. (1997) *Towards equality: A Christian manifesto*, London: SPCK.

Holman, B. (1998) *Child care revisited: The Children's Departments 1948-1971*, London: Institute of Child Care and Social Education.

Holman, B. (1999) 'A voice from the estate', in S. Timms, G. Dale, H. Stanton and B. Holman, *Joined-up writing: New Labour and social inclusion*, London: Christian Socialist Movement.

Holman, B. (2000) *Kids at the door revisited*, Lyme Regis: Russell House Publishing.

Holman, B., Carol, Bill, Erica, Anita, Denise, Penny and Cynthia (1998) *Faith in the poor*, Oxford: Lion Publishing.

Home Office (1998) *Supporting families*, London: The Stationery Office.

Home Office, Ministry of Health and Ministry of Education (1946) *The report of the care of children committee* (Curtis Report), London: HMSO.

Home Office, Ministry of Education and Science, Ministry of Housing and Local Government and Ministry of Health (1968) *Report of the committee on local authority and allied personal social services* (Seebohm Report), London: HMSO.

House of Commons (1984) *Second report from the social services committee: Session 1983-84, Children in care*, London: HMSO.

Hutton, W. (2000) 'The economics of poverty', in A. Carpenter, R. Nicholson and D. Robinson (eds) *What if?*, London: The Short Book Company.

Issacs, S. (ed) (1941) *The Cambridge evacuation survey*, London: Methuen.

Jacobs, M. (1995, reprinted 1998) *D. W. Winnicott*, London: Sage Publications.

Jervis, M. (1987) 'The man who founded his own branch of social work', *Social Work Today*, 2 February.

Jones, C. (2001) 'Working for the welfare', 18th Duncan Memorial Lecture, Liverpool: University of Liverpool.

Jordan, B. (2000) *Social work and the Third Way*, London: Sage Publications.

Kahan, B. (1949) *Report of the first year of the Children's Department 1948-1949*, Dudley: Dudley Children's Department.

Kahan, B. (1970) 'The child care service', in P. Townsend, A. Sinfield, B. Kahan, P. Mittler, H. Rose, M. Meacher, J. Agate, T. Lynes and D. Bull, *The fifth social service*, London: Fabian Society.

Kahan, B. (1980) *Growing up in care*, Oxford: Blackwell.

Kahan, B. (ed) (1994) *Growing up in groups*, London: HMSO.

Kahan, B. (1999) 'Child care through the ages', *Community Care*, 4-10 November.

Kahan, B. and Levy, A. (1991) *The Pindown experience and the protection of children*, Staffordshire: Staffordshire County Council.

Kanter, J. (undated) *Clare Winnicott: Her life and legacy*, Maryland: unpublished [note: some of the material in this unpublished draft later appeared in Kanter, J. (2000) 'The untold story of Clare and Donald Winnicott: how social work influenced modern psychoanalysis', *Clinical Social Work Journal*, vol 28, no 3, pp 245-61].

Kelly, G. (1998) 'The influence of research on child care policy and practice', in D. Iwaniec and J. Pinkerton (eds) *Making research work*, Chichester: Wiley.

Land, H. (1985) 'The introduction of family allowances: an act of historic justice?', in C. Ungerson (ed) *Women and social policy*, London: Macmillan.

Land, H. (1990) 'Eleanor Rathbone and the economy of the family', in H. Smith (ed) *British feminism in the twentieth century*, Aldershot: Edward Elgar.

Lawrence, F. (2001) 'Mass affluents get richer as the new poor get poorer', *The Guardian*, 2 April.

Lewis, J. (1983) 'Eleanor Rathbone and the family', *New Society*, 27 January.

Lowe, R. (1995) 'The rediscovery of poverty and the creation of the Child Poverty Action Group', *Contemporary Record*, vol 9, no 3, pp 602-9.

Lowe, R. and Nicholson, P. (1995) 'The formation of the Child Poverty Action Group', *Contemporary Record*, vol 9, no 3, pp 612-27.

Macnicol, J. (1980) *The movement for family allowances 1918-1945*, London: Heinemann.

Marwick, A. (1964) *Clifford Allen: The open conspirator*, Edinburgh and London: Oliver and Boyd.

Marwick, A. (1976) *The home front*, Edinburgh and London: Thames and Hudson.

Maureen (1971) 'Killing the poor', *New Society*, 25 November.

Ministry of Health (1944) *Hostels for 'difficult' children*, London: HMSO.

Morgan, K. (1990) *The people's peace: British history 1945-1989*, Oxford: Oxford University Press.

Murphy, J. (1992) *British social services: The Scottish dimension*, Edinburgh: Scottish Academic Press.

National Association for Mental Health (1946) *Report of child guidance inter-clinic conference*, London, November.

NISW (National Institute for Social Work) (1982) *Social workers: Their role and tasks* (Barclay Report), London: Bedford Square Press.

ONS (Office for National Statistics) (1998) *Social Trends Quarterly*, London: The Stationery Office.

ONS (1999) *Social Trends 29*, London: The Stationery Office.

Packman, J. (1975) *The child's generation*, Oxford and London: Blackwell and Robertson.

Parker, H. (ed) (1998) *Low cost but acceptable: A minimum income standard for the UK: Families with young children*, Bristol: The Policy Press.

Parker, R. (1966) *Decision in child care*, London: Allen and Unwin.

Parker, R. (1980) *Caring for separated children*, Basingstoke: Macmillan Press.

Parker, R. (ed) (1999) *Adoption now: Messages from research*, Chichester: Wiley.

Paxman, J. (1991) *Friends in high places: Who rules Britain?*, London: Penguin.

Pederson, S. (1996) 'Rathbone and daughter: feminism and the father at the fin-de-siecle', *Journal of Victorian Culture*, vol 1, no 1, pp 98-117.

Philpot, T. (1977) 'Championing the children's cause', *Community Care*, 7-13 September.

Rathbone, E. (1903) *Conditions of labour at the Liverpool Docks*, Liverpool: private.

Rathbone, E. (1905) *William Rathbone: A memoir*, London: Macmillan.

Rathbone, E. (1909) *How the casual labourer lives*, Liverpool: Liverpool Women's Industrial Council.

Rathbone, E. (1924) *The disinherited family*, London: Edward Arnold.

Rathbone, E. (1940) *The case for family allowances*, London: Penguin.

Residential Child Care Association, Association of Children's Officers and Association of Child Care Officers (1968) *The residential task in child care* (Castle Priory Report), London: Residential Child Care Association.

Rowe, J. and Lambert, L. (1973) *Children who wait*, London: Association of British Adoption Agencies.

Rowntree, B.S. (1901) *Poverty: A study of town life*, London: Macmillan (reissued by The Policy Press/Joseph Rountree Foundation, 2000).

Rowntree, B.S. (1941) *Poverty and progress*, London: Longmans.

Rowntree, B.S. and Lavers, G. (1951) *Poverty and the welfare state*, London: Longmans.

Scottish Home Department (1946) *Report of the committee on homeless children* (Clyde Report), Edinburgh: HMSO.

Secretary of State for Social Security (1999) *Opportunity for all: Tackling poverty and social exclusion*, London: The Stationery Office.

Shaw, M., Dorling, D., Gordon, D., and Davey Smith, G. (1999) *The widening gap: Health inequalities and policy in Britain*, Bristol: The Policy Press.

Shearer, A. (1970) 'Government clashes with poor group', *The Guardian*, 20 April.

Simey, M. (1974) *Eleanor Rathbone 1872-1946: A centenary tribute*, Liverpool: Liverpool University Press.

Sinfield, A. (1969) *Which way for social work?*, London: Fabian Society.

Social Exclusion Unit (2001) *A new commitment to neighbourhood renewal: National strategy action plan*, London: Cabinet Office.

Stocks, M. (1949) *Eleanor Rathbone*, London: Gollancz.

Stocks, M. (1970) *My commonplace book*, London: Peter Davies.

Stroud, J. (undated) *Memoirs of John Stroud*, Hertfordshire: private.

Stroud, J. (1960) *The shorn lamb*, London: Longmans Green.

Stroud, J. (1961a) *On the loose*, London: Longmans Green.

Stroud, J. (1961b) *Touch and go*, London: Longmans Green.

Stroud, J. (1965) *Labour of love*, London: Longmans Green.

Stroud, J. (1968) *Up and down the city road*, London: Hodder and Stoughton.

Stroud, J. (1971) *13 penny stamps*, London: Hodder and Stoughton.

Stroud, J. (ed) (1973) *Services for children and their families: Aspects of child care for social workers*, Oxford: Pergamon Press.

Stroud, J. (1988) 'That stroke of mine', Hertfordshire: unpublished.

Stroud, J. (1989) 'Poems', Hertfordshire: unpublished.

Temple, W. (1942) *Christianity and social order*, London: Penguin.

Thomas, J. (1970) 'Preface', in *ACCO commemorative report 1949-1970*, London: ACCO.

Thompson, P. (1999) *Peter Townsend: Life story interview*, Colchester: University of Essex.

Thorpe, D. (1994) *Evaluating child protection*, Buckingham: Open University Press.

Townsend, P. (1952) *Poverty: Ten years after Beveridge*, London: PEP.

Townsend, P. (1957) *The family life of old people*, London: Routledge and Kegan Paul.

Townsend, P. (1958) 'A society for people', in N. Mackenzie (ed) *Conviction*, London: MacGibbon and Kee.

Townsend, P. (1962a) *The last refuge*, London: Routledge and Kegan Paul.

Townsend, P. (1962b) 'The meaning of poverty', *The British Journal of Sociology*, vol 13, no 3, pp 210-27.

Townsend, P. (ed) (1972) *Labour and inequality*, London: Fabian Society.

Townsend, P. (1973) *The social minority*, London: Allen Lane.

Townsend, P. (1979) *Poverty in the United Kingdom*, London: Allen Lane and Penguin.

Townsend, P. (1993) *The international analysis of poverty*, Hemel Hempstead: Wheatsheaf.

Townsend, P. and Davidson, N. (1982) *Inequalities in health: The Black Report*, Harmondsworth: Penguin Books.

Townsend, P., Corrigan, P. and Kowarzik, U. (1987) *Poverty and labour in London*, London: Low Pay Unit.

Townsend, P., Leith, P., Tumin, Sir S. and Verma, J. (1996) *The great, the good and the dispossessed*, London: Channel 4 Television.

Townsend, P., Sinfield, A., Kahan, B., Mittler, P., Rose, H., Meacher, M., Agate, J., Lynes, T. and Bull, D. (1970) *The fifth social service*, London: Fabian Society.

Toye, A. (1970) 'The launching', in *ACCO commemorative report 1949-1970*, London: ACCO.

Tunstill, J. (ed) (1999) *Children and the state: Whose problem?*, London: Cassell.

Van Dijken, S. (1998) *John Bowlby: His early life*, London: Free Association Books.

Weinstein, E. (1960) *The self-image of the foster child*, New York, NY: Russell Sage Foundation.

Whelan, R. (1996) *The corrosion of charity*, London: Institute of Economic Affairs.

Wilkinson, R. (1994) *Unfair shares*, Barkingside: Barnardo's.

Wilkinson, R. (1996) *Unhealthy societies*, London: Routledge and Kegan Paul.

Wilson, H. (1962) *Delinquency and child neglect*, London: Allen and Unwin.

Wilson, H. and Herbert, G. (1978) *Parents and children in the inner city*, London: Routledge and Kegan Paul.

Winnicott, C. (1964) 'Casework and agency function', in C. Winnicott, *Child care and social work*, Hertfordshire: Codicote Press, pp 59-70.

Winnicott, C. (1970) 'A toast to ACCO', in *ACCO commemorative report 1949-1970*, London: ACCO.

Winnicott, C. (1st edn, 1984, 2nd edn, 1995, reprinted 1997) 'Introduction', in C. Winnicott, R. Shepherd and M. Davis, *Deprivation and delinquency: D.W. Winnicott*, London: Routledge.

Winnicott, D. and Britton, C. (1947) 'Residential management as treatment for difficult children', *Human Relations*, vol 1, no 1, pp 2-12.

Women's Group on Public Welfare (1943) *Our towns: A close-up*, London: Oxford University Press.

Index